The Jossey-Bass Health Series brings together the most current information and ideas in health care from the leaders in the field. Titles from the Jossey-Bass Health Series include these essential health care resources:

At Risk in America: The Health and Health Care Needs of Vulnerable Populations in the United States, Lu Ann Aday

Changing the U.S. Health System: Key Issues in Health Services, Policy, and Management, Second Edition, Ronald M. Andersen, Thomas H. Rice, Gerald F. Kominski, Editors

Collaborating to Improve Community Health: Workbook and Guide to Best Practices in Creating Healthier Communities and Populations, Kathryn Johnson, Wynne Grossman, Anne Cassidy, Editors

Competitive Managed Care: The Emerging Health Care System, John D. Wilkerson, Kelly J. Devers, Ruth S. Givens, Editors

Critical Issues in Public Health, C. Everett Koop, Editor

Curing Health Care: New Strategies for Quality Improvement, Donald M. Berwick, A. Blanton Godfrey, Jane Roessner

Designing Health Care for Populations, Applied Epidemiology in Health Care Administration, Peter J. Fos, David J. Fine

Health Care 2010: The Forecast, The Challenge, Institute for the Future

Health Care in the New Millennium: Vision, Values, and Leadership, Ian Morrison

Immigrant Women's Health: Problems and Solutions, Elizabeth J. Kramer, Susan L. Ivey, Yu-Wen Ying, Editors

Managed Care in the Inner City: The Uncertain Promise for Providers, Plans, and Communities, Dennis P. Andrulis, Betsy Carrier

New Rules: Regulation, Markets, and the Quality of American Health Care, Troyen A. Brennan, Donald M. Berwick

People in Crisis: Clinical and Public Health Perspectives, Second Edition, Lee Ann Hoff

Raising Standards in American Health Care: Best People, Best Practices, Best Results, V. Clayton Sherman

Regulating Managed Care: Theory, Practice, and Future Options, Stuart H. Altman, Uwe E. Reinhardt, David Schactman, Editors

Remaking Health Care in America (Second Edition)*: The Evolution of Organized Delivery Systems,* Stephen M. Shortell, Robin R. Gillies, David A. Anderson, Karen Morgan

To Improve Health and Health Care: The Robert Wood Johnson Foundation Anthology, Stephen L. Isaacs, James R. Knickman, Editors

Trust Matters: New Directions in Health Care Leadership, Michael H. Annison, Dan S. Wilford

Oxymorons

Oxymorons

The Myth of a U.S. Health Care System

J . D . K L E I N K E

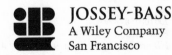

JOSSEY-BASS
A Wiley Company
San Francisco

Published by

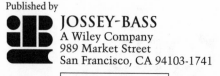

JOSSEY-BASS
A Wiley Company
989 Market Street
San Francisco, CA 94103-1741

www.josseybass.com

Jossey-Bass books and products are available through most bookstores. To contact Jossey-Bass directly, call (888) 378-2537, fax to (800) 605-2665, or visit our website at www.josseybass.com.

Substantial discounts on bulk quantities of Jossey-Bass books are available to corporations, professional associations, and other organizations. For details and discount information, contact the special sales department at Jossey-Bass.

We at Jossey-Bass strive to use the most environmentally sensitive paper stocks available to us. Our publications are printed on acid-free recycled stock whenever possible, and our paper always meets or exceeds minimum GPO and EPA requirements.

Library of Congress Cataloging-in-Publication Data
Kleinke, J. D.
Oxymorons: the myth of a U.S. health care system / J.D. Kleinke.
p.; cm.—(The Jossey-Bass health series)
Includes bibliographical references and index.
ISBN 0-7879-5970-7 (alk. paper)
1. Medical care—United States. 2. Medical policy—United
States. 3. Health care reform—United States.
[DNLM: 1. Managed Care Programs—trends—United States. 2.
Health Care Reform—United States. W 130 AA1 K64o 2001] I.
Title. II. Series.
RA445 .K56 2001
362.1'0973—dc21
2001004587
First Edition
HB Printing   10 9 8 7 6 5 4 3

CONTENTS

PREFACE

I contradict myself? So then,
I contradict myself.

Walt Whitman

One of the strengths of the Internet is also one of its great cruelties: it remembers everything. The Web site for *The Newshour with Jim Lehrer* on PBS includes a transcript of my effusive commentary, dated April 2, 1996, on the $8.8 billion merger between Aetna and U.S. Healthcare into a massive health insurer with 23 million members.

"The managed care revolution has brought to health care a much more organized, rational way of delivering health care," I told the cameras. "HMOs and other kinds of managed care companies seek to improve your health status and prevent disease progression, while steering you toward physicians who have better demonstrated quality."

I was a true believer in the managed care revolution, and I could scarcely contain my enthusiasm about what this merger meant for those 23 million people. I believed in the promise of managed care and expressed that belief openly and passionately on national TV, in the editorial pages of the *Wall Street Journal* and *JAMA,* and in my 1998 book *Bleeding Edge: The Business of Health Care in the New Century* (Kleinke, 1998a). I argued that the economic and organizational disciplines unleashed by HMOs like U.S. Healthcare were harsh but necessary medicine for the systemic illnesses that have afflicted the financing and delivery of health care in the United States since the emergence of modern medicine. I was convinced (and occasionally convincing) that the consolidation of hundreds of fragmented health plans across the country meant economies of scale, lower administrative costs per member, and broader access to disease management systems that would improve the collective health of the insured population.

I also staked my career on it. During the 1990s, I helped build a company, HCIA, that bet more than half a billion dollars in Wall Street money on the boldest promises of managed care. We created and sold information products designed to help the U.S. health care system fix itself. Those of us who worked or invested in the health care information industry believed that under the prodding of managed care, hospitals and physician organizations would finally be forced to embrace the information revolution that had been transforming the rest of the economy for more than a decade. Our efforts helped form the very fabric of the managed care movement; the products and systems we built were designed to improve the quality and lower the cost of medical care through the standardization, measurement, and analysis of patient and provider data.

My bubbling enthusiasm for the Aetna–U.S. Healthcare merger evaporated in less than two years, when several dozen physician colleagues and friends faxed me a form letter sent by the newly merged health plan to every major physician organization in California. The letter declared that Aetna U.S. Healthcare would no longer negotiate payment rates or enter into contracts with those physician organizations, most of which were formed specifically to negotiate managed care contracts on behalf of busy physicians in small group practices. With a combined 23 million insured lives as a bargaining chip, the new corporation was using a divide-and-conquer strategy. The doctors—even those "with better demonstrated quality"— were on their own.

Of course, Aetna U.S. Healthcare eventually reaped what it sowed: its wholesale bullying of provider organizations backfired when a handful with sufficient market presence or power (for example, the Mayo Clinic) publicly canceled contracts with the massive insurer. The public relations fallout that followed both underscored and complicated Aetna's mushrooming operational and financial problems. Since the merger, the company has been singled out for special vilification in the trenches, as reflected in numerous conversations with physician friends and colleagues; many report that they go out of their way to tell their patients to avoid the insurer whenever possible. Once again, 23 million human bargaining chips are caught in a game of marketplace poker created by managed care in which everybody ultimately loses.

Five hard years after the Aetna–U.S. Healthcare merger, conventional wisdom has it that managed care has failed to live up to all but its most brutal promises. Left in the rubble are bewildered consumers, disappointed employers, enraged patients, embittered physicians, and a raft of lawsuits—along with a handful of failed or enfeebled health care information vendors. What once looked like a permanent reduction in health insurance premiums—thanks to a onetime round of severe price competition among managed care organizations—turned out to be an anomaly, a momentary pause in their inevitable rise. And the overwhelming majority of clinical studies have shown that for all their rhetoric about population health, illness prevention, and disease management, managed care systems do not improve the overall health status of their members. In the final analysis, most "managed care" really was "managed cost" all along—but it failed to accomplish even that goal, and the U.S. health care system is worse off for the experiment.

Although it is easy and occasionally fun to pick on the bad manners and various hypocrisies of managed care, it is also unfair. The nation's managed care organizations were asked to do a job that simply cannot be done. Out of our collective naivete and idealism, we did not know this at the time. As a society, we expected managed care to fix, in a few short years, the disaster in slow motion that is the U.S. health care system. We asked large, organizationally complex insurance companies to reform a century's worth of self-serving professional habits, rein in ever-expanding consumer and patient demands, and fix dysfunctional economic behaviors—all while answering to the taskmasters on Wall Street every quarter. Mindful of the waste and inefficiency choking our medical system, we were certain that managed care could simultaneously reduce costs and improve quality. And painfully aware of the runaway costs associated with poorly managed diseases, most of us believed that these insurance companies could do well financially by doing good medically. We were wrong.

An abiding faith that free-market principles would fix the U.S. health system—as seen in the nation's rejection of the Clinton reform plan, employers' whirlwind love affair with managed care, and my own book *Bleeding Edge*—grossly underestimated three simple, intractable facts about the financing and delivery of medical care in this country. First, chaos is the rule in the delivery of medicine, not an aberration of the rule. Second, behavioral inertia among the dozens of layers of health care administration wrapped around the actual delivery of medicine is the inevitable consequence of the first fact. And third, most executives, consultants, pundits, and other thought leaders in health care have so discounted the power and durability of the first two facts that they are prone to repeating the same beliefs—regardless of how erroneous or silly—until everybody else believes them: *physician risk-contracting will fix everything, consumerism will fix everything, employer coalitions will fix everything, "leadership" will fix everything, the Internet will fix everything.* As of this writing, the health care twaddle du jour has it that defined contribution–style health benefits will fix everything.

Throughout this book I refer to these three intertwined and implacable facts of health care life as, respectively, our system's Chaos Factor, Inertia Factor, and Twaddle Echo Factor. Collectively, these three forces represent a death sentence for almost any fix for what ails the U.S. health care system, be it a private market initiative or act of public legislation. Every "solution" an entrepreneur or politician can dream up runs headlong into the utter complexity of the system, the uncanny ability of those working in it to defend their precious turf against the solution, and the constant disconnect between what people in health care say they are going to do and what they actually end up doing. This is nobody's fault. It is the fault of a badly broken system. As Deming observed in *Out of the Crisis*—his 1982 landmark study of industrial engineering that inspired the quality movement in American business—it is wrong to blame individuals for bad outcomes when they are producing those outcomes in a bad system.

Doctors, hospitals, managed care executives, drug companies, patients, consumers, employers, entrepreneurs, and every other economic agent in health care are all trying to manage their way through the chaos of the system as they find it—and in the process are making that chaos even worse. This is why I have dedicated Chapter Five of this book to an exploration of chaos theory in the context of both medicine and health care. If we fully understood chaos theory and its terrifying implications for our industry, or acknowledged the pervasive inertia that comes in response to that chaos, or recognized our own unwitting echoing of the latest twaddle about how to rid the system of both, we would be far less cocksure about promoting the newest unworkably complex business strategy, however fashionable. Such strategies are peddled across the country in waves by the nation's consulting companies. They fail soon after the consulting and legal bills are paid. And then the next generation of surefire "solutions" plays the health care conference circuit. The only things that change are the names of the hot new health care companies and the themes of the conferences.

Consider one of the great clichés mouthed at these conferences: the only constant in health care is change. I would revise this bit of warhorse of punditry by arguing, with some bitterness, that the only constant in health care is the anxious anticipation of change that never actually occurs. By 1998, it was assumed by all that capitation would replace fee-for-service reimbursement across the United States in a few short years. The promise of capitation was the subject of more than a dozen books, its clinical and economic power was quantified in several compelling studies in the peer-reviewed literature, and it served as the inspiration for countless new and retooled consulting businesses. The financial discipline and administrative elegance of paying provider groups a lump sum for a healthy patient—rather than line item by line item, when that patient fell ill—were too compelling for the market not to adopt capitation universally, as provider groups grew sophisticated enough to manage themselves under the new payment system. Oops! Capitation failed before it ever really got a chance to take hold. Why? For three reasons. First, it was sold by insurers in bad faith (that is, with inadequate dollars and insufficient supporting data) as an economic quick fix for busy people who never fully understood its implications and were organizationally unprepared to manage its complexities. Second, institutional and economic inertia made true capitation impossible to implement. And finally, the next round of twaddle was quick to explain away capitation's failure before it had a chance to work. As the medical director of a physicians' group explained, "We have three systems of compensation: the one we used last year, the one we are using this year, and the one we will use next year" (Bodenheimer and Casalino, 1999). I would venture to say that the compensation system that group will use two years from now will be the same one they used last year. After ten years of expensive flirtation with risk-based provider contracting, "discounted" fee for service remains the dominant payment mechanism across the U.S. health care system, and all the well-documented market failures associated with fee-for-service medicine continue. The long view of our industry's history shows that health care is not changing so much as running in place, faster and faster, consuming more and more dollars as it tries to "reengineer" itself out of its own realities.

If we are ever going to think our way out of this mess, we need to take a fearless look at both its origins and most truculent features. This may be the ideal time for just such a look, as we seem to be taking a momentary breather from the numbing repetition of marketplace fixes and near-instantaneous failures that characterized health care throughout the 1990s. The year is 2001: the managed care revolution has failed, most of the physician practice management companies are in ruins, the conquest for national domination of the hospital market by Columbia-HCA has been broken by the government, and drug companies are under attack, once again, for making money on the backs of sick people. As of this writing, some of the loudest contributors to the Twaddle Echo Factor have become uncharacteristically circumspect, if not altogether mute. We are engulfed in a sort of Ecclesiastes phase of health care, where the greatest minds seem capable only of ever more incisively articulating the hopelessness of the problem.

So too, this book. Consider yourself forewarned: the goal of *Oxymorons* is to take an unsentimental, unflinching look at the tortuous history and implacable dynamics of health care in America, to find in that history and those dynamics some guideposts for what we can reasonably expect the marketplace to fix, and to propose broad regulatory solutions for those things we should no longer expect the marketplace to fix, informed as we are by more than a decade of its desperate and often destructive attempts to do so.

The first seven chapters take you on a dark, discomfiting journey through the worst architectural features of the colossal mess we call a health care "system" in this country. The objective is to tear apart the entire accidental nondesign of this nonsystem to see (1) how health care in the United States came to be so broken; (2) which parts of the nonsystem are worth preserving and protecting; and (3) which parts are the biggest troublemakers that should be pulled out and discarded so the whole thing will work better. The goal of Chapter Eight is to propose a set of simple but sweeping reforms that the federal government can undertake to accomplish exactly this. Finally, because the overriding tone of *Oxymorons* is politically impassioned, emotionally unvarnished, and admittedly vitriolic, the ninth and final chapter is my own story—a narration of the odyssey that has informed and inspired my deepest beliefs about what is best and worst about the U.S. health care system. Yes, too many otherwise rational debates about health care are derailed by personal anecdote, but because so many colleagues and readers have inquired about the real source of my politics and passions on the subject, I thought a coda to *Oxymorons* would be the ideal way to put my own anecdote down for the record, once and forever.

This, like everything else about *Oxymorons*, is an enormous departure for me. *Bleeding Edge* was an unapologetic championing of market forces in the U.S. health care system. For years I was one of the many who believed and argued that health care organizations of all kinds could do well financially by doing good medically. One of my best friends, former health care journalist Craig Havighurst, was extremely critical of *Bleeding Edge's* almost libertarian embrace of market-based reform and its willful disregard of the problem of the uninsured. That omission was no accident; the goal of the book was to show health care providers how to cope with the various disciplines introduced into the system by managed care. In that regard, I believe the book was useful and still is. But helping providers and others cope with an inherently broken system does nothing to fix that system.

I believed when I wrote *Bleeding Edge*—and believe still—that most Americans do not want a single-payer, government-run system. We want a health care system financed by private insurance, delivered by lots of competing providers, and driven by personal choices. And we are reaching a new boiling point as the baby boom generation approaches an outdated Medicare system with great trepidation and an unwillingness to compromise personal medical demands for lower collective health care costs.

If anything, the legislative reforms at the heart of *Oxymorons* will promote an even greater reliance on real market forces in the U.S. health care system. The purpose of this book is to focus on the market imperfections and resulting organizational clutter that hamper, complicate, and often cripple (at least for the uninsured) the financing and delivery of health care in the United States, much of which flows from the result of a few unfortunate accidents of our social and political history.

Fasten your seat belt. You are in for a rough ride.

J.D. Kleinke

Clear Creek County, Colorado

July 2001

ACKNOWLEDGMENTS

Because there is no boundary between my work and my life, my most trusted professional colleagues are also my closest personal friends. Without them, this book, the career that informs it, and the life that has inspired it would be barren and joyless.

Kathleen Ford sustains me professionally. Over the years, she has been a diligent research assistant, copy editor, graphic designer, detail-monger, reality check, and hassle filter. Joshua Blum, M.D., is my medical collaborator and conscience. He has happily sullied many a good bike ride and mountain climb to parse an important clinical point or illuminate a health care theory with a medical example; his own commitment to both medicine and patient care resonates through all of my work. Andrew Pasternack, my editor at Jossey-Bass, helped conceive, give birth to, and nurture this book. What you have in hand is as much a product of Andy's encouragement as it is one of my own efforts.

I would also like to acknowledge others instrumental in the literal and spiritual shaping of this book: Genevieve Bell for her graciousness; Eric Berger for his love of sensible health policy; Elizabeth Berger, M.D., for her sensitivity; Marc Berger, M.D., for his wry intelligence; Robert Bodner for his brotherhood; Robert Brook, M.D., for his unflinching intellectual drive; Brian Buchanan for his patience; John Cook III, M.D., for his mentoring on chaos theory; Michael Dalby for his business wisdom; Sharon Engkvist for her spirit; Mary Jane England, M.D., for her insights; Andrew Essreg for reminding me that it would still be snowing in the backcountry when

I finished this book; Wendy Everett for her integrity; Alexander Ford for his wit; Rachel Gaffney, M.D., for her smile; Sheila Fifer for her enthusiasm; Katherine Goodman for her steadfastness; Craig Havighurst for his many passions; Karen Hedman for her artistry; John Iglehart for his championing; Patrick Jeffries for his irony; Jody Kennedy for her political passions; Leonard Kish for his raw lay intelligence; Allan Khoury, M.D., for his unshakable faith in what is still possible; Scott Leibowitz, M.D., for his humor; Meg Lemon, M.D., for her enormous heart; Sarah Loughran for her energy; Donald Metz for his precision; Julie Moran for her laughter; David and Jane Perkins for their friendship; George Pillari for his uniquely pragmatic literacy; Uwe Reinhardt for his candor; Sean Riley for his intensity; Mara Rubin for her strength; Quenton Stricklin for his dedication to the cause; Deborah Tolman for her nurturing; Nancy Mari Watson, J.D., for her vigilance; Archibald Warnock for his skepticism; Karen Williams for her good cheer; Christine Yang, M.D., for her daily if unseen presence in my life; and Andrea Zuercher for her linguistic purity.

I would like to thank the dozens of writers, editors, and staff members of *Health Affairs, JAMA, The New England Journal of Medicine, Managed Healthcare Executive, Modern Healthcare,* and the *Wall Street Journal* who have assisted me over the years both directly and indirectly. Their diligence, commitment, and sacrifices have provided substance and inspiration to all of my work.

ABOUT THE AUTHOR

J.D. Kleinke is president and CEO of HSN, a medical software development company based in Colorado. He is the former vice president of corporate development for HCIA Inc., a pioneering health care information company. From 1992 through 1998, he helped lead HCIA from start-up data analysis firm to publicly traded provider of health care information systems and products with $80 million in annual revenues. Before joining HCIA, Kleinke was director of corporate programs at Sheppard Pratt Health System, the largest private psychiatric hospital in the United States. While at Sheppard Pratt, he developed and managed the nation's first provider-based managed mental health care system. Kleinke's work has been published in the *Wall Street Journal, JAMA, Health Affairs, Barron's,* the *British Medical Journal,* and *Modern Healthcare.* He is a director of several health information technology companies, a member of the editorial board of *Health Affairs,* and author of the book *Bleeding Edge: The Business of Health Care in the New Century.* He holds an M.S.B. in finance from Johns Hopkins University and a B.S. in economics from the University of Maryland.

For my sister, Betsy,
for teaching me the most important things

*Medicine's role is to entertain us
while Nature takes its course.*

Voltaire

CHAPTER 1

Wars, Strikes, Riots, and Acts of Congress

I n 1943, at the height of World War II, a forty-eight-year-old shipyard laborer had a major heart attack, spent a week in the hospital, and was unable to return to work for two months. His wife and teenage son both worked at the same shipyard, and begged the boss for extra pay to help cover the family's medical bills. Though the boss was sympathetic to their situation and wanted to increase their wages, he could not because of a new law freezing wartime pay—a law designed to control inflation during a period of scarce labor and round-the-clock work schedules.

He gazed out his office window, through the sparks and smoke and dust of the bustling shipyard, and spotted the big white hospital on the horizon, a long bus ride away for his workers.

Why not pay the hospital directly myself? he wondered. They get their raise, the guy gets his bills paid, and I'm still right with the law. Better yet, why not bring some of those doctors over here to the shipyard? They can take care of these people in that empty office downstairs. That way, they don't lose so many hours from the yard when they need something checked. How hard can that be? How much can it possibly cost?

There is no U.S. health care system. What we call our health care system is, in daily practice, a hodgepodge of historic legacies, philosophical conflicts, and competing economic schemes. Health care in America combines the tortured, politicized complexity of the U.S. tax code with a cacophony of intractable political, cultural, and religious debates about personal rights and responsibilities. Every time policymakers, corporate health benefits purchasers, or entrepreneurs try to fix something in our health care system, they run smack into its central reality: the primary producers and consumers of medical care are uniquely, stubbornly self-serving as they chew through vast sums of other people's money. Doctors and hospitals stumble their way through irresolvable conflicts between personal gain and ethical responsibilities; patients struggle with the acrimony and anguish that accompany life-and-death medical decisions; consumers, paying for the most part with everybody's money but their own, demand that the system serve them with the immediacy and flexibility of other industries; and health insurers are trapped in the middle, trying to keep everybody happy. A group of highly imaginative, energetic people armed with the world's largest Mark-n-Wipe board could not purposefully design a more complex, dysfunctional system if they tried. It is a $1.3 trillion per year fiasco narrated with moral shrillness and played out one competing anecdote after another.

A bustling shipyard may not be the best place to receive our medical care, but in spirit, that is where most of us with commercial insurance get it. Because of a unique and difficult moment in our nation's history, our health care system was slapped on top of our employment system, with the government picking up the enormous slack for most of those who fell outside that system. And so it began. The imposition of the nation's employers, insurance companies, legislators, lawyers, investment bankers, insurance brokers, and countless other corporate and regulatory middlemen into the financing and delivery of medical care is the source of the fundamental structural problems that cripple health care in this country. The endless layering of interloper upon interloper—all ultimately charged with managing the shipyard's or the government's money—dooms the market's ability to fix any of the system's root problems.

The best proof of how impossible it is to rationalize the spending of $1.3 trillion every year is the twisted set of paradoxes at the heart of the managed care industry. Managed care as we know it consumes an ever larger share of money earmarked for medical care, in the process replacing the chronic disorganization of American medicine with acute overorganization. Managed care has added more layers of complexity and redundancy to the financing and delivery of medical care, solving none of its underlying economic dilemmas while introducing a new set of political, cultural, and behavioral problems. If managed care provides us with one overriding message, it is this: the U.S. health care system as currently structured is so complicated and rife with economic conflict that every attempt to simplify it actually complicates it further.

THE ACCIDENTAL PATIENT

The U.S. health care system grew out of a series of historical accidents. Today, most commercially insured Americans receive their health care coverage through their jobs or unions. This is a legacy of our metaphorical shipyard boss's attempt to cope with the economic struggles created by World War II. Those who retire from the shipyard, are fired, cannot get hired, or end up permanently disabled all count on a combination of federal and state government agencies for help. The unlucky 44 million Americans caught in the middle—in the no-man's land outside of good jobs, union membership, major disability, old age, or chronic poverty—have no coverage at all, fending for themselves in a system built to accommodate everyone else. Contrary to popular belief, those 44 million uninsured do in fact receive medical care. But they get it only when their medical conditions have deteriorated to the point of crisis, at unnecessarily great expense to themselves, to taxpayers, to those working in the shipyard, and to their own already marginal personal solvency.

During the wage freeze necessitated by the labor shortage of the 1940s' wartime economy, employers across the nation began adding health coverage as a noncash incentive to attract and retain scarce workers. Their successful lobbying of Congress for a tax exemption for this compensation created a permanent cultural expectation that health insurance be not only free, but tax-free. Under employer-based insurance, every time a worker demands a medical service paid for directly or indirectly by his employer, he is, in effect, giving himself a tax-exempt raise. The economic and behavioral effects of this system are deeply perverse and go a long way in explaining why the United States spends far more per capita on medical care than any other nation in the world. Tax-free, job-based insurance—combined with mushrooming consumer medical information and advertising— induces people to demand more medical care than they would if they were spending their own hard-earned, highly taxed income. It also creates a shadow, regressive tax system, whereby the best compensated employees are encouraged to demand still more health benefits rather than cash to escape marginal taxation on this compensation. In the metaphorical shipyard, the temptation to drop your tools and go see the "free" doctor—at any time, for any reason—is often overwhelming.

Employers have responded to this dysfunctional system by giving freely with one hand while attempting to manage what they give with the other. The dirtiest work associated with managing what is perceived by employees as free has been delegated by employers to health insurers, brokers, consultants, and myriad other third, fourth, fifth, and sixth parties. The cumulative result is mistrust, misunderstanding, bitterness, reactive legislation, and lawsuits; complex gamesmanship throughout the dysfunctional "love triangle" of purchasers, patients, and their doctors; and an ever-growing thicket of paperwork surrounding the whole mess.

The clearly capitalist thrust of job-based—that is, merit-based—health insurance grated on the social architects of the Great Society, who sought to fill the gaps by providing equivalent benefits to the elderly and poor through the creation of Medicare and Medicaid in the 1960s. Because of the historic, ongoing struggle between federalism and states' rights, those architects decided that the financing of Medicare should be the responsibility of the federal government; the administration of Medicare should be the work of the states; half the financing of Medicaid should be the responsibility of the federal government, with the other half the responsibility of the states; and the administration of Medicaid should be the full responsibility of the states. The resulting schizophrenic provision of what

4

should be a uniform public benefit has resulted in total confusion over which level of government pays for what medical care and why, a bewildering array of financial transfers and a political cat-and-mouse game between the states and Washington, and a mother lode of bureaucratic complexity.

As if inspired by the inefficiencies and uncertainties created by a combination of state and federal administration of public health care benefits, the government inadvertently extended the benefits of this same system to the nation's employers through another legislative accident. Since the passage of the McCarran-Ferguson Act in 1945, private health insurance plans have been regulated by the states. Under this law, fifty different states were required to build fifty different regulatory systems for overseeing premiums, mandating levels of coverage, and disciplining health insurers—even though most Americans receive their coverage from health insurers who operate across state lines and in many cases across the entire country. Fair enough. Even as small companies grew and merged into large national corporations over the past few decades, with employees scattered across dozens of states, this may have made sense given the uniquely local nature of medical care delivery, economics, and abuses.

But then another legislative earthquake erupted. In 1974, the federal government passed the Employee Retirement Income Security Act (ERISA), designed to protect retirees' pension funds in states without sufficient regulatory oversight. It created provisions under which the boss in the shipyard could self-fund his workers' pension plans, established uniform standards for that self-funding, and strengthened federal insurance protections in case the shipyard went bankrupt and could not pay out those pensions. ERISA also happened to contain a "minor" provision that extended the new law to cover those few, large national employers who chose to self-fund their health benefits as well as their pension plans. Duke University health law professor Clark Havighurst points out that "ERISA was enacted in response to some highly publicized instances of fraud and mismanagement with respect to pension funds and was not perceived by Congress as a health care measure at all" (Havighurst, 2000).

As companies like the shipyard grew in size, added or acquired workers across the country, and chafed at the regulations imposed willy-nilly on their health benefit plans across fifty different states, many of them took advantage of the ERISA exemption. Meanwhile, medium-size employers, in response to the same state-based regulatory burdens, also chose to self-insure under ERISA. As a result, one-third of privately insured people today have health coverage regulated by the federal government, whereas two-thirds have health coverage regulated by their states. Aside from a few seemingly arbitrary mandates imposed by new federal laws—and the passage in 1996 of one long overdue federal law regarding health insurance portability—55 million insured Americans receive whatever specific health benefits their employers choose to cover (Wechsler, 2000). The other 105 million privately insured, employed Americans receive a set of highly defined benefits depending on the state they live in, and their employers are forced to pay for them. Neither system works well, and the combination of the two systems attempting to work in parallel creates an administrative fiasco for health insurers that has drained billions of health insurance dollars otherwise earmarked for medical care.

"How much can it possibly cost?" our shipyard boss wondered, back in 1943. Little did he know that much of what he would end up paying for decades later would have nothing to do with medical care for his shipyard workers, and everything to do with how big the shipyard grew, where it chose to do business, how its workers voted, and how many lawyers set up shop down the street.

THE ACCIDENTAL PROVIDER

Meanwhile, over the decades, what has happened to the big white hospital across town and the doctor in the office downstairs? They too have expanded what they do and where, in the process coping with their own series of historic and legal accidents.

If the demand side of the health care equation is checkered with a complex series of accidental, often unintelligible variables, the supply side of the equation is just as complicated. Specific supply-side variables driven by health policy accidents include, but are certainly not limited to, the following:

- Conflicting ownership and management of different kinds of U.S. hospitals, depending on state laws
- Tortured relationships between U.S. hospitals and the physicians who drive their costs and business fortunes
- A series of cynical, poorly thought-out laws on the financial relationships of physicians and hospitals
- Complicated legal relationships among physicians themselves when they attempt to negotiate their own business fortunes with everyone from the metaphorical shipyard to the various middlemen negotiating on its behalf

With the backdrop of these institutionalized economic, cultural, and philosophical conflicts—and the occasionally bizarre public policy or application by the courts of unrelated legal precedent—is it any wonder that even the most earnest entrepreneurial attempts to make a health care business work do not go according to plan?

Attempts throughout the 1990s to "integrate" the delivery of health care—among physician groups and between physician groups and hospitals—have been complicated by a set of laws passed nearly a century ago. The ownership of physician practices is governed by ridiculously antiquated laws still on the books in numerous states (but not all states) against the so-called corporate practice of medicine. This archaic legal doctrine, fashionable in state legislatures in the 1920s, was designed to prevent financial considerations from affecting clinical decision making. (The long view of history frequently allows us a good laugh at the naivete of earlier generations, embodied in so many attempts over the years to legislate away normal human behavior.) If our shipyard operates in a corporate-practice-of-medicine state, then it cannot directly employ the doctor downstairs but it can enter into an exclusive business contract that carries few of the advantages and most of the drawbacks of direct employment. Across town at the hospital, the same corporate-practice-of-medicine law makes the already complicated task of building an integrated delivery system a legal circus. Because it is technically illegal for hospitals or other corporations to own physician practices outright, the laws have compelled the creation of additional corporate structures on top of existing physician and hospital corporate structures.

The result is a set of health care organizations that resemble Chinese boxes—organizations within organizations within organizations, each with their own legal ownership, governance boards, officers, managers, and financial records. The situation benefits no one, except perhaps the armies of lawyers who happily churn their way through all the resulting paperwork on a billable hourly basis. Health care contracting dollars that flow from a self-insured employer like our shipyard to the actual caregivers in the innermost box pass from that employer through an alphabet soup, including the national TPA (third-party administrator), the local TPA, the MSO (management services organization), the IPA (independent practice association), and finally the PA (professional association or corporation) that actually employs the physicians. Each acronym represents a tollbooth along the way, taking a piece of the care dollar and contributing greatly to the Chaos Factor that employers, consumers, and patients confront when they attempt to navigate the system. Each acronym also adds to the Inertia Factor, which hampers those employers or coalitions of consumers that—when dissatisfied with some dimension of the care process—try to simplify administrative procedures, suggest clinical reform, or introduce a disease prevention or management initiative.

IS THERE A DOCTOR IN THE CORPORATION?

That is the mess we make when we try to integrate physicians and hospitals at the legal and corporate levels. Making it actually work is another story altogether. Lawyers may be deft at creating an ever-expanding number of corporate shells around hospitals and their admitting physicians, but they cannot make the people working inside those shells get along. In health care, the same cultural diversity that makes America such an adaptive, vibrant

8

nation is a significant impediment to the system's progress. This cultural diversity is manifested in the wide variety of hospital ownership and management patterns across the country, which range from fiercely not-for-profit hospital organizations—both sprawling and small—run by very different religious organizations, to for-profit hospital organizations both large and small run by entrepreneurs with very different goals and philosophies, to large medical centers with rich academic cultures and an exotic mix of foreign-born professionals.

Historically, U.S. hospitals have been "self-ghettoized" by their religious affiliation, or in the absence of any religious affiliation other than fealty to the almighty dollar, by their tax status. As Paul Starr notes in his brilliant, durable book *The Social Transformation of American Medicine,* "Cultural heterogeneity has been one of the chief factors inhibiting consolidation of hospitals in a state-run system. Ethnic and religious groups have wanted to protect their own separate interests" (Starr, 1982, p. 176). This situation is not unique to the U.S. system. Medical sociologist and historian William Glaser noted that around the world, "The greater the number of religions in a society, the more diffused the ownership and management of hospitals and the smaller their average size" (p. 176). As the most heterogeneous of the world's leading nations, the United States suffers from the worst diffusion and complexity of hospital ownership and management. This historic truth about our cultural diversity does much to explain the U.S. health care system's enormous fragmentation when compared with the rest of the world. Attempts since the late 1980s to consolidate different hospitals in a community based on market need have run headlong into inevitable cultural and philosophical conflicts as they try to mix nuns on a mission to serve the poor with corporate managers on a mission to serve their shareholders.

These are the obvious problems to anticipate and manage. More insidious cultural and economic conflicts arise inside the walls of an individual hospital. A principle struggle in hospital management has always been the constant complicating factor of the de facto veto power by a hospital's nonemployees over nearly every aspect of its day-to-day operations. Indeed, physicians drive the bulk of a hospital's costs and exercise control over nearly all of its actual employees but have no real vested interest in its success. The Medicare system galvanized the historic economic and operational disunion between hospitals and physicians by replicating and expanding what was already an antiquated schism. With the rise of the early "Blues" plans in the 1930s and 1940s, insurance for hospital care and physician services was financed and managed by separate organizations: Blue Cross versus Blue Shield. Thanks to more rational alternatives offered by integrated insurance plans like Kaiser Foundation Health Plan and Group Health of Puget Sound, this system was just starting to wither when Medicare was created. However, the architects of the program enshrined this split when they created Medicare's own payment system in the 1960s. This split still runs down the middle of the Medicare system today, no matter how silly and counterproductive it appears to even the most casual observer. Because of this fault line between payment systems, hospitals and physicians function at economic cross-purposes. Lump-sum Medicare Part A payment compels hospitals to speed up the discharge of patients, whereas line-item-by-line-item Part B payment compels physician specialists to slow them down. More chaos, more inertia.

The legal and financial disunion between the hospital across town and the admitting colleagues of the physician downstairs in our metaphoric shipyard has always subjected hospitals to the vagaries of physician clinical decision making. This disunion has left them vulnerable—in the worst case scenario—to economic recklessness and substandard clinical practices. Traditionally, however, the disunion between hospitals and physicians did not matter. Before managed care, when all patients wielded blank checks written on the shipyard's account, sloppy physician practices made more money for the hospital. After all, substandard medical care or surgical technique—when it does not kill patients or entice malpractice attorneys—will almost always result in longer stays, more drugs, longer detours through the ICU, and bigger bills.

Managed care screwed all that up. When our shipyard boss started to discover just how much his vision back in 1943 was costing him by the mid-1980s, he took drastic action. He hired a new kind of third party, a managed care organization (MCO), to keep tabs on exactly what the hospital across town was doing and what it was charging him for it. He also asked the MCO to keep an eye on what the doctor downstairs, whom he could not legally employ or control, was doing and charging for it.

Through the 1990s, the price pressures of consolidating MCOs compelled hospitals to seek closer economic alignment with, and some might say greater business control over, their admitting physicians. This made sense economically *and* clinically, and it was one of the few signs that the economic disciplines of managed care really did hold promise for improving the way medical care was organized and delivered. Throughout the 1990s, consultants went into overdrive working on reimbursement and compensation models that pursued these alignments. Thanks to the Twaddle Echo Factor, everybody became convinced that in a few short years these models would come to redefine the entire medical care landscape, and every freestanding hospital and group of physicians would be happily engaged in a contractual, if not corporate, version of the vertical integration of a Kaiser or Group Health.

But just as managed care was taking hold, the federal government went and screwed *that* up. The historic disunion between hospital services—the highest cost component of health care—and all those physicians driving most of those services has been reinforced by what are commonly known as the Stark laws. In the mid-1990s, Congressman Fortney "Pete" Stark (D-California) championed two incredibly complex Medicare-related payment laws that have foiled all meaningful attempts to integrate what doctors do with what hospitals need them to do. Combined with similar so-called anti-kickback laws passed a few years earlier, the Stark anti-self-referral laws have foiled numerous efforts to integrate doctors and hospitals over the past ten years. These laws have grossly complicated every attempt to align hospitals and physicians economically, most glaringly the gain-sharing arrangements that would have rewarded legally independent physicians for helping hospitals manage inpatient costs more efficiently ("HMOs," 1999).

Attempts to comply with these laws—which stem from the presumption that most U.S. physicians are thieves who cannot be trusted with the blank checks handed over by Medicare beneficiaries—have forced hospitals and physician groups to create still more corporate layers for the simple purpose of joint contracting with health plans for insured populations. They have also forced those within the corporate layers to seek "safe harbors" from subsequent prosecution by submitting details of their business plans to the Justice Department. The department reviews the plans for months and then, if it approves them, publishes the details for all to see (with the corporate names removed) as so-called advisory opinions. As a result of this process, if a hospital simply wants to pay a doctor an extra thousand dollars for a good surgical outcome or faster discharge of patients from its ICU, it needs to get what amounts to a proactive legal settlement. Not quite an act of Congress, but the next best thing. Once again, this is a boon for the lawyers, a headache for the busy health care executive, more costs for our metaphorical shipyard to bear, and an economic drag on the entire U.S. health care system. Let us pretend for a moment that these laws did not exist. In their absence, whatever fraud and waste we as taxpayers would endure from truly self-dealing physicians and hospitals could not possibly outweigh the costs of the gross operational inefficiencies associated with economically disenfranchised physicians, not to mention the costs when thousands of hospitals are forced into protracted legal compliance rituals with each attempt at an innovative hospital-physician integration strategy.

Of all the legal accidents that have complicated or even doomed well-meaning attempts by providers to fix the health care delivery system, none is more paradoxical than the antitrust rulings as they relate to physicians. In 1975, the Supreme Court ruled in *Goldfarb* v. *Virginia State Bar* that the "learned professions" are engaged in "trade or commerce" and therefore are not exempt from antitrust actions when they attempt to band together for the purposes of collective negotiation of their own payment rates. The ruling meant that although consolidating health insurers can impose payment rates on physicians, the physicians cannot stand together to push back. The Twaddle Echo Factor has it—erroneously, judging from physician pricing data from across the country—that the *Goldfarb* ruling galvanized competitive market forces in the fragmented physician community. Many also believe that it paved the way for the consumerism that will prove to be the panacea for what ails the U.S. health care economy.

Goldfarb has become the cornerstone of physician antitrust law. Based on this precedent, physicians are free to charge as little or as much as they want, independent of each other, and attempts to do otherwise open them up to possible antitrust actions. But in actual practice, *Goldfarb* makes contract-based integration of fragmented physician practices tortuous and uncertain. After a decade of twaddle about "care integration," physicians are still forced, even with safe-harbor protections, either to risk prosecution, collude in secret, or go it alone against well-organized health insurers, running the business of their practices the way they always have—in legal, commercial, and clinical isolation.

The doctor practicing downstairs in the shipyard is thus left legally and financially defenseless against the new MCO hired by the boss. It is not a fair fight. Finally, there is a supreme irony in the *Goldfarb* case. Just like ERISA, it had nothing to do with health care—it was an antitrust case against the legal profession.

A MEDICAL CHICKEN IN EVERY POT?

Much of the U.S. health system's complexity arises from its hybrid private and public funding. *This* is no accident. The shipyard worker's health care is paid for by the boss, and the worker has very clear and growing expectations of what that means. His retired neighbor, covered by Medicare, has the exact same expectations. Both want to go to the "best" hospital in town, see their own doctor, and have access to the same new medicines. When one falls ill, gets a certain level of medical care, and tells the neighbor about it, the other's expectations are raised accordingly.

The uneasy coexistence of public and private health insurance systems in this country reflects our deeply rooted cultural conflict about medical care, one that is unique in the industrialized world. Is access to the best medicine a basic human right or an earned privilege? The answer to this question depends on whom you ask. As a society we are incapable of deciding, so we decide by not deciding. This indecision becomes even more entrenched when we add the issue of specific level and caliber of medicine to which American citizens either have a basic right or must earn the privilege as workers and taxpayers. How else can you explain why the chronically poor, infirm elderly, and prison population often have access to state-of-the-art surgical and drug therapies, while a steadily employed blue-collar worker who cannot afford health insurance has access to nothing except the emergency room?

This is the health care edition of the split Congress, the traditional chocolate versus vanilla politics of American life that forces us into electoral choices that most of us do not want to make. As a culture of ambitious shipyard employees, we are philosophically split between the personal drive to get rich quick and a populist sympathy for the oppressed worker. Yet we are trapped into choosing: between the Democrats' self-serving faith in bureaucracy-expanding "compassion" for the disenfranchised and the Republicans' self-serving fealty to lower taxes and the resulting "opportunity" that lower taxes supposedly create, if only for those already benefiting from opportunities harvested by their parents. Our ambivalence over whether every U.S. citizen is entitled to the best medical care in the world, or should be forced to earn that entitlement, pervades all political debate on the subject and has always precluded the creation of coherent, bipartisan health policies that have any chance of actually working.

In everything but health care, we resolve this conflict with bare-bones solutions and trickles of money per disenfranchisee. Not counting the de facto welfare programs administered by the defense and agriculture departments, our housing, food stamp, school lunch, and other welfare programs provide a thin safety net for only the most marginalized of American people. In health care, by contrast, this safety net has expanded to cover nearly half the population—if you define the safety net as the combination of official government programs for selected groups, with the "system" of cross-subsidies, hospital tax breaks, foundation-funded clinics, medical residency funding, and drug company largesse that provide care for the uninsured (Fronstin and Helman, 2000).

The philosophical impasse over the nature of medical care entitlement in America, propagated in shipyard worker neighborhoods across the United States, serves as yet another fault line, this one running through the center of every one of our health care institutions. It not only affects but often dominates policy debates over everything from the financing of physician education, to the regulation of commercial MCOs, to the amount of charity care provided by hospitals, to the future of the Medicare and Medicaid programs. As of this writing, the public financing of prescription coverage for Medicare beneficiaries is stumbling over precisely this fundamental philosophical impasse. Should seniors have unlimited, publicly funded access to the entire pharmaceutical arsenal? Should they have such access only to those drugs that are critical to saving their lives rather than improving the quality of those lives? Or should they make this decision for themselves, in the marketplace, with a combination of government funding and their own money?

The cultural and philosophical ambivalence about our rights to medical care in this country has turned the financing and management of the Medicare and Medicaid programs into a fifty-one-ring circus. Those in Congress who believe the government can fix everything want to expand these programs to include more segments of American society, one group at a time; those on the other side of the aisle want to go in the opposite direction and fully privatize both programs. As a result, neither side prevails, and these enormous, already complex programs grow by inches into an ever more multidimensional hybrid of expanding government agencies, nonprofit organizations, and for-profit companies. Roughly 15 percent of Medicare beneficiaries have their care administered by private MCOs; the rest have their care administered by a crazy quilt of federal contractors. As a result, who pays a Medicare beneficiary's different medical bills can vary not only within the same community, or even family, but for that same beneficiary, depending on which type of care she received and from whom. The enrollment choice she may have made the previous fall is only one of several variables. Similarly, the Medicaid program in many states is run by the state government, the same program in other states is run by nongovernmental nonprofit agencies, and the same program in still other states has been handed over to one or more for-profit HMOs. In all three cases, the actual medical care is delivered by both for-profit and nonprofit providers. The Chaos Factor that pervades this system when viewed across the country ensures that the Inertia Factor will preclude any meaningful, systemic reform.

By the mid-1990s, momentum was building for a greater share of these public programs to convert to private programs. The commercial supporters of such privatization, making good use of the Twaddle Echo Factor, argued that consolidating, competing MCOs created economic efficiency and better customer service systems, which in turn presented attractive alternatives to the traditional Medicare and Medicaid programs. Why this turned out to be pure twaddle and never coalesced depends, once again, on whom you ask. The MCOs claim that the government underpaid them, they were never able to make money, and they were thus forced to restrict what they could offer. According to the American Association of Health Plans (AAHP), more than half of all commercial health insurers lost money on Medicare risk contracting because of underpayment (conversation with AAHP spokesperson, June 20, 2001). In contrast, the government claims that the insurers never achieved the efficiencies they claimed they could and thus could not make money on legislated prices that were more than adequate. According to a Justice Department audit, Medicare overpaid managed-care companies by $1.8 billion in fiscal year 2000 (Taylor, 2000). Here's where the Twaddle Echo Factor gets really interesting. Conservative conspiracy theorists believe the Clinton administration kept those prices artificially low on purpose, setting up the whole privatization movement to fail and leading to a subsequent expansion of government management. Liberals see the Medicare risk-contracting meltdown as sweet vindication, launching into the familiar chorus that there is something evil, or at least unsavory, about trying to profit from the delivery of medical care to sick people—the insurers got what they deserved.

The truth, as in most things involving a struggle for the soul of health care in America, has little to do with these polarized philosophies. All the managed care rhetoric notwithstanding, MCOs are unable to earn profits on fixed price contracts with the government for the simple reason that

16

more stuff cannot be provided for less money. Under managed-care risk contracting for Medicare beneficiaries, the federal government paid 88 cents on the traditional fee-for-service dollar. For this shrunken benefit dollar, the health plans were expected to provide *more* benefits, cover their added marketing and administrative costs, and make a profit. This is the something-for-nothing accounting that made the Clinton reform plan the laughingstock of the health insurance lobby and those in Congress who helped defeat it. As Chapter Three will explore at length, the fundamental premise of managed care is flawed. Forget the Twaddle Echo Factor about proactive prevention and disease management saving money. The MCOs were doomed from the start when they set out to make money with their more-for-less market offerings to elderly consumers and patients who will always demand more. When the shipyard worker tells his bald neighbor in a Medicare HMO about a great new drug that is helping a bald guy at work, what is the neighbor's obvious response?

If government-dictated prices for Medicare beneficiaries do not work, why do we not have competitive bidding for those beneficiaries by for-profit MCOs, the same way we have supposedly competitive bidding for military work by for-profit defense contractors? We have been trying to move toward exactly this kind of system since the mid-1990s, and it has been a resounding failure. The MCOs argue that the "competitive pricing demonstration" process, attempted for years to no avail, has set them up to fail; the government argues back that the MCOs do not really want to compete; the nation's providers blame everybody for excluding them from the process; and consumer activists think the whole process is evil. And so it goes. An astute summation of the problem can be found in a preface to an edition of *Health Affairs* that included hundreds of pages of research on the failure of Medicare to create a competitive managed care pricing project. "No single culprit is to blame, because every interest involved had a hand in derailing this effort" ("Painful Pursuit," 2000, p. 6).

The numerous irreconcilables that cripple the debate over how much to pay an MCO to take care of the shipyard worker's bald neighbor—a highly demanding beneficiary of a public entitlement program—is one more variation on our broader theme. What should be a simple analysis of medical cost allocations and normal rates of return for the delivery of a public service has tumbled headlong into the same old muck. Is medical care a market good that is subject to market prices or a special human right that should be sacrosanct?

Our cultural ambivalence over this problem, applied only recently to health insurers, has been a permanent feature of the provider financing landscape for decades. How much to pay hospitals and doctors who treat Medicare and Medicaid beneficiaries is one of the most complicated and costly annual rituals in Washington, as the federal government seeks to legislate a set of prices affecting nearly $400 billion in annual spending—prices that also end up as reference points for much of the private sector. As a result, the business fortunes of hospitals, physician specialties, and other types of providers rise and fall at the whim of government reimbursement policies. When hospitals make too little money at something, they lobby Congress for payment increases. When they make too much, a Congressional "watchdog" or member of one of several regulatory agencies charged with overseeing health care smells a rat and attacks. The clearest example of this process was the nearly five-year persecution of the once-ambitious hospital company, Columbia-HCA, by the Justice Department for various business, administrative, and accounting practices. Under its founder and former CEO Richard Scott, Columbia was enormously successful at playing by the arbitrary legal and reimbursement rules created by the federal government, and making money. Columbia was seen as a growth stock on Wall Street, a favorite with mainstream and aggressive mutual fund managers alike, which gave the company a fat currency for expanding its unapologetically for-profit health care empire. This resulted in a highly publicized witch-hunt, the ouster of Scott and his lieutenants, the makeover of the company by less aggressive, more conciliatory executives, and a record $840-million fine (Taylor, 2001). Five years after the dramatic, symbolic raid on Columbia's first hospital by gun-toting federal agents, the company has shrunk to two-thirds its original size and been renamed "HCA, The Healthcare Company." The message of the Columbia scandal to hospitals is clear: you can make money on the backs of Medicare patients, but God help you if you make too much and brag about it to Wall Street.

18

I'M FROM THE GOVERNMENT, AND I'M HERE TO AUDIT YOU

In its funding of health care entitlement programs, the government, like employers, gives with one hand and takes away with the other. With government driving nearly half of health care purchasing in the United States, the provider community is vulnerable, year by year, to the whimsy of public policy, which echoes every subtle change in the perennial emotional debate over the essential nature of medical care entitlement. U.S. hospitals spent fifteen years learning to cope with the introduction of lump-sum DRG payments for Medicare inpatients, rationalizing their operations to weed out excess costs and sloppy care patterns built up over the previous decades. Then in 1997, with one stroke of the legislative pen, nearly the entire hospital industry's profitability—built up through this process—was torn down by the Balanced Budget Act. By 1998, the impact of the government's attempts to manage the entire federal budget by starving the nation's hospitals was starting to show (Jaklevic, 2000b).

This reversal of fortune reversed again in 2000, when hospital lobbyists convinced Congress of the damage the Balanced Budget Act had done. The highest monthly increase in hospital revenues since 1995 occurred in October 2000, exactly one month after the rollback (Bellandi, 2000b). And so, although hospitals should be focused on putting their houses in order, they spend the balance of their time and energy coping with how that house measures up to the government standards of the day. These standards change drastically with every new presidential administration; they also change more subtly, every two years, with shifts in the balance of power in Congress.

Although the winds of political change distract and distort the normal functioning of the typical U.S. hospital, the problem is especially ferocious for the hundreds of teaching hospitals across the country, which conduct some of the most important work in the health care system. Under a hybrid private and public health care system, teaching hospitals have conflicted missions. They receive extra public funding to conduct research, train doctors, and care for the uninsured, but they also seek to compete in the commercial marketplace with nonteaching hospitals, despite the economic and organizational burdens associated with their other noncommercial activities. As a result, hospitals affiliated with academic medical centers carry a 20 to 30 percent surcharge over nonteaching hospitals. Researchers have found that roughly half this surcharge is funded by the federal government and the rest comes from higher prices in the commercial market. "Considerable uncertainty exists about the reliability of [the federal government as] funding source in the future," those researchers note in *Health Affairs*. "Higher payments from multiple private-sector insurers have been a more reliable source of revenues" (Anderson, Greenberg, and Lisk, 1999, p. 164). For now, this means that the "brand" value of a teaching hospital in its community—and the public's perception that this brand value translates into better care—is all that sustains that hospital as a business. It is a testament to the business skills of those running these institutions that they are able to convey the value of that brand, while coping with the pricing pressures of managed care and simultaneously dealing with all the politics and economics attendant to a reliance on government funding.

Teaching hospitals are remarkably adept at coping with a central fact about health care in the United States: under hybrid public-private financing of medical care, our system, though driven by common consumer expectations fostered by neighbors sharing their medical experiences, is really three completely different systems, all running in parallel. One system exists for those with a public entitlement, another for those with private insurance, and still another for those with neither. The splintering of the system into three parallel systems has trained providers to cope as best they can, forcing them to choose, independent of actual clinical need, which patients get what care, when, and for how much. Providers charge completely separate sets of prices for patients with identical conditions. They are coerced economically into treating those identical conditions differently, in accordance with completely different types of coverage rules. And then they are held accountable for variations in the care they deliver. The cumulative result of this system is the persistence of distinct patterns of medical technology diffusion and utilization. The demand side of the health care equation, bolstered by neighborhood discussions across the country and a wealth of health information provided by the media, grows rapidly and rather harmoniously; the supply side does not.

Small wonder that decades of research have shown one stubborn feature about medical care in America: the kind of care you receive in this country has less to do with how sick you are and more to do with the kind of health insurance you carry. If the MCO hired to manage the shipyard's medical costs is especially tightfisted, the worker may have no access to a needed diagnostic procedure, whereas his neighbor covered by Medicare will get the same procedure every year. Throughout the medical literature, we see patterns of care that vary as much by insurance status as by age, sex, and race. Such variations provide the perfect rationale for the government's strategy of "managing" the care it delivers by policing the provider community for compliance with its reimbursement rules. It does not help that such compliance must occur in accordance with a reimbursement rulebook that is forty-five thousand pages long and counting, nor that all the laws against self-referral are so vague that they are useless without extensive, preemptive legal documentation. This rulebook is the manifestation of the Chaos Factor in the health care system, and obsessive attempts to comply with it give rise to much of the system's Inertia Factor—an often insurmountable hurdle for numerous well-meaning attempts at innovation by providers.

The federal government's efforts to root out and penalize providers for failure to comply with these rules, known collectively as acts of fraud and abuse, accomplish two things: they serve as a de facto rebate program for a fraction of the $400 billion it spends on medical care; they also ape the IRS's strategy of using the fear of reprisal to compel voluntary compliance among providers when seeking government reimbursement. A public flogging in the pages of *Modern Healthcare,* the *Wall Street Journal,* and a provider's hometown newspaper signals to all providers in the community that anything but the most conservative interpretation of the rules contained in those forty-five thousand pages will result in prosecution, professional disgrace, and financial ruin.

Thus providers seeking to make money on delivering health care to those with a public entitlement do so at the risk of being branded criminals when their navigation of the system slips past a set of invisible tolerances. As Havighurst observes, the "government has found it convenient to characterize provider conduct that exploits the program's shortcomings as 'fraud and abuse' and to criminalize it. The moral spin was necessary to overcome the presumption that all providers are entitled to participate in Medicare and to shift responsibility for the program's deficiencies away from its designers" (Havighurst, 2000, p. 90). Through the detection and prosecution of this so-called fraud and abuse, the government is in effect admitting that it cannot proactively manage its own purchases. It overpays and then goes after a portion of that overpayment, a bizarre process that seeks a tortuous equilibrium between provider profiteering and insolvency. Such is the endgame of using private organizations to deliver a public good for the one-third of the American citizenry that consumes one-half of all health care costs.

BACK ALLEYS AND "INTEGRATED" CARE SYSTEMS

The many bitter conflicts attendant to delivering a public good through private means grow especially shrill and emotional in the arena of reproductive health care. Because the issue of reproductive freedom will come up throughout this book, let me state my moral and political position on this subject once and for all. Voluntary abortions may be morally repugnant, but they are far less repugnant than the words and actions of those with the audacity to judge, legislate, or otherwise interfere in this most sacred, profound, and personal of human choices. I am not an advocate of abortion. I am, however, an advocate of fully preserving the awesome, terrible responsibility that the Supreme Court has guaranteed American women. And I stand in vehement opposition to anyone who—frustrated by both the Supreme Court's guarantee and the large majority of Americans who support abortion rights—resorts to acts of domestic terrorism and harassment of patients, physicians, and their families to achieve what their political meddling cannot. Regardless of one's own personal position on the subject, the impact of this bitter, permanent philosophical debate on the politics of the U.S. health care system is the same: when we use public money to finance private medical choices, we run into enormous trouble.

Over the past decade, as hospitals around the United States have struggled to integrate their fragmented operations into "systems" of care, our national stalemate over reproductive health almost always rears its ugly head. In many cases, it derails an entire hospital integration effort, even though reproductive health represents a tiny fraction of the total package of services involved. A good example is the protracted legal and political wrangling within the BayCare Health System in Florida, which controls approximately half the hospital beds in the Tampa–St. Petersburg area. The BayCare system includes several Catholic hospitals, which like most (but not all) Catholic hospitals have refused to coordinate their services with other BayCare hospitals that provide the full range of women's health services, including surgical sterilization and abortion. One of the key hospitals in the system, Bayfront Medical Center, sits on land leased by the local government. Consistent with constitutional law that (generally) guarantees the separation of church and state, the city insisted that Bayfront not acquiesce to its Catholic partners and continue to provide the full range of women's health services. Making the BayCare system comply with constitutional doctrine would clearly put it into conflict with Catholic doctrine. The system spent nearly $1 million in legal fees trying to sort through the mess before finally giving up. According to a report in *Modern Healthcare*, members of the eight-hospital system kicked Bayfront Medical out because neither the hospital nor the system could "continue to justify a costly legal battle with the city" (Bellandi, 2000a, p. 24).

This drama plays itself out in communities across the country, often to very different ends. Some systems accommodate their Catholic partners in often bizarre ways; others dig in their heels. How shrill does the screaming over this issue get? When Frances Kissling, president of the lobbying group Catholics for a Free Choice, spoke out against the rollback of reproductive services in hospital alliances between Catholic and non-Catholic hospitals, a "pro-life" group issued a press release calling her an "ex-Catholic" and a "heretic." Luckily for Kissling, those seeking to follow up on their medieval condemnation of her would have trouble finding her street address because the group spelled her name incorrectly in the press release ("Outliers," 2001). The acrimony of this debate and the plurality of its resolution in different communities is a testament to the widespread governance and internal struggles of the Catholic church, the heterogeneity of the U.S. health care system, and to our point, the hazards of mixing public money with private health care systems.

This local drama also plays itself out at the national level in the nearly perennial debate over changes to the financing of Medicaid and Medicare coverage. Antichoice lawmakers use the public funding of private health care choices by the poor and disabled as a way of advancing their broader political agenda. The result is that those women in the United States with the most desperate economic and personal need for access to the full array of reproductive choices have those choices placed in the greatest jeopardy. Like all political struggles over abortion rights, and all struggles over medical care entitlement, the more vulnerable you are, the fewer options you get.

CHOCOLATE AND VANILLA POLITICS

I have no faith that we as a society will ever resolve the abortion rights debate or any other philosophical conflict attendant to the public financing of private health care choices. We remain a nation of Democrats and Republicans, of staunchly pro-choice and antichoice voters, of hardworking taxpayers and needy entitlement beneficiaries who will never agree on the most fundamental of all health care questions: Is access to everything our medical community has to offer a basic human right or a hard-won privilege? The best we can do is acknowledge the implacability of this debate and the plurality it represents. We should create health care reform policies that acknowledge and accommodate this, and leave the rest to be sorted out in the marketplace.

Such an accommodation is a key element of the reform plan outlined in Chapter Eight of this book, the one dedicated to tax parity. Because government pays for nearly half of all medical services in the United States, we have decided one thing: health care is a social good, and an investment in our collective health status is worthwhile at the most fundamental level. The shipyard boss inadvertently made this determination back in 1943 when he chose to pay for his workers' medical care and bring a doctor into the workplace. Our desire to pay for better medical care with tax-free dollars—and tax dollars themselves—is a central tenet of American public health policy and social beliefs; it provides a rationale for the continued tax deductibility of health insurance premiums and other expenses for those fortunate enough to have job-based health benefits.

The biggest problem arises when the shipyard boss—fed up with high costs and the failure of the MCO he hired to managed those costs—stops paying for his workers' medical care. The shipyard worker is then forced to fend for himself, going without insurance or trying to buy it on the retail market with aftertax dollars. All other pricing matters being equal (and they are not), the same medical coverage and care that cost the shipyard 75 cents will cost the worker on his own a full dollar in pretax income. This is wrong.

If, as a society, we believe that Americans should have unlimited access to all the medical care they need, want, and can afford, then we should remove the tax distortions that give one group of Americans this access while restricting it for another group. Such tax parity will finally help remove the complexity and conflicts created by the imposition of employers into the health care system while accommodating two central beliefs about health care in this country: Americans should be entitled to unlimited access to whatever medical care they can afford and are willing to pay for, and they should do so through the private marketplace.

CHAPTER 2

Playing with the Boss's Money

Jim and Dave, two men in their midthirties who met during a bank management seminar, are having a beer after a Saturday afternoon of golf. Jim works for a large national bank company headquartered on the East Coast; Dave works for a locally owned bank. They are both branch managers, and though they would sooner discuss their sex problems than disclose their incomes to each other, they make exactly the same salary. As usual, the subject turns to Dave's kids.

After boasting about his son's latest swim meet, Dave asks Jim, "So when are you and Jenny taking the plunge?"

With hesitation, Jim reveals his and Jenny's difficulty conceiving a child. They have been trying for years, both have been tested by their doctors, and it turns out that Jenny has a fertility problem. It can be overcome, but only with a treatment regimen that costs $10,000 and does not guarantee results.

"So?" Dave asks. "Our insurance covers it. Go for it!"

"No, it doesn't," Jim says.

"Sure it does."

"I thought you had PrimeCare? That's what we have at our bank," Jim says. "We checked, and the fertility treatment isn't covered."

"Sure it is," Dave insists, reaching for his wallet and pulling out his insurance card. "We have PrimeCare. And a woman who works for me had that done last year, all fully paid for after her deductible. She ended up having twins."

Jim reaches for his wallet and pulls out his insurance card. It is identical to Dave's, except for the group number and policy number.

On Monday morning, Jim's wife Jenny checks with PrimeCare one more time, armed with the new information. After four phone transfers and sitting on hold for fifteen minutes, she is told one more time that in vitro fertilization (IVF) is not covered by her plan and never has been. According to the member services representative at PrimeCare, the woman who works with Dave in the local bank was probably covered because she is in PrimeCare's "fully insured fiduciary product governed by last year's IVF state mandate."

As discussed in Chapter One, the imposition of the nation's employers into the U.S. health care system is a legacy of World War II. The first HMO was a product of this same twist of fate: the Kaiser Health Plan began as a prepaid set of clinics and hospitals surrounding the shipyards of Henry J. Kaiser, one of the war's largest contractors (Starr, 1982). This isolated moment in history has flourished over the decades into the ever-expanding miasma of complexity, inefficiency, mistrust, legal conflict, and unintelligible telephone explanations that define today's employer-based private health insurance system. The tax deductibility of the premiums paid by the two banks that employ Jim and Dave—a significant financial benefit unavailable to consumers buying their own insurance on the open market—perpetuates this accident of history and its many unintended consequences. At last count, employers were financing medical care for their employees to the tune of more than $300 billion per year (Sheils and Hogan, 1999).

Under this system, the typical insured American has been acculturated over the decades to understand—as in Jim's exhortation to "Go for it!"— that every time he demands more expensive medical care, he is giving himself, in effect, a tax-free raise. But these tax-free raises are not free. They translate directly into diverted cash compensation, which helps explain both the acute stagnation in personal income during periods of high medical cost inflation and the chronic decline in health insurance coverage during those same years. According to a study in *Health Affairs,* "Decline in health insurance coverage among workers from 1979 to 1995 can be accounted for almost entirely by the fact that per capita health care spending rose much more rapidly than personal income during this time period" (Kronick and Gilmer, 1999, p. 31).

With $300 billion of their own money at stake, U.S. employers are forced to micromanage our health care system. They either do so on their own—if reluctantly and usually poorly—or outsource the effort to health insurers to do so on their behalf. In perennial debates in statehouses across the country, where legislatures create new laws requiring health insurers to provide specific benefits to their covered members, those employers who do not self-fund their benefits under ERISA tend to default to the political positions taken by health insurers on these mandates. Specifically, they lobby against medical services—such as IVF for women like Jenny—that they do not want to be forced by their host state to cover. In general, larger employers who *do* self-fund under ERISA—to our point, Jim's bank—are free from these state-level mandates. At the same time, they are forced to side with smaller employers like Dave's bank and the health insurers in lobbying against a whole separate set of federal benefit mandates.

The political face of employers is greatly at odds with the one they show to all the Jims and Daves they employ. Although lobbying against benefit mandates protects the employer's financial interests at the potential expense of its employees' health, the employer still tends to cave in to employee pressure on benefit design. (Imagine Jim or Dave organizing their coworkers to agitate for IVF coverage from the banks that employ them.) Even after joining with the insurers to succeed in killing a mandate in a state legislature, the employer will then turn around and force its contracted health insurers to pay for those very same benefits, often benefits that the plan itself may not value or want to provide. (This may have happened at Dave's bank, had the IVF mandate not been passed by the state legislature.)

This situation—along with much of what is wrong about an employer-based health insurance system to begin with—is made worse because the purchasing of health coverage is usually managed by corporate human resource departments. Human resource departments, aside from being among the weakest parts of most corporations, tend to focus on providing benefits and keeping employees happy rather than on the real value of specific benefits like IVF, which are negatives from a financial perspective. This exacerbates the fundamental problem of employment-based health coverage, "in which benefits are highly visible and costs are not." This, according to Havighurst, "helped to breed the pervasive entitlement mentality that still distorts political discussions about health care. Today's backlash against managed care owes a lot to working Americans' ability to see only the possible drawbacks of their new coverage and not the substantial savings that managed care has added to their paychecks" (Havighurst, 2000, p. 88).

TEN THOUSAND LITTLE HEALTH CARE SYSTEMS

In attempting to manage their way through this unmanageable situation, every major U.S. employer has, in effect, created its own U.S. health care system in miniature. The employer decides which services, drugs, types of providers, and other resources are covered, and for whatever medical necessity it deems severe enough. In so doing, employers like Jim's bank are forcing their own values and choices, many of which are highly moralistic, on millions of Jims and Jennys. Conservative companies will not pay for the full spectrum of reproductive services; sexist companies will pay for vasectomies but not birth control pills; progressive companies will extend health coverage to unmarried domestic partners and pay for less traditional treatment alternatives, many of which, ironically, are actually more cost-effective, including nurse-midwives for childbirth and hospices for end-of-life care. These choices are the employers' right to exercise. It's their money, their workplace, and their values. And at least in theory, Jim is perfectly free to join or leave the company as he sees fit. But it is a stupid system, and all new hires must beware.

As an illustration of just how stupid this system is, consider the following questions, which are based on recent stories in the popular press describing the struggle of employers to work through some life-or-death health benefits debates:

30

- Just how bad does an employee's allergies have to be before he or she is entitled to a prescription antihistamine?
- Is this worker's husband really worried about benign enlargement of his prostate—or losing his hair?
- Does a male-to-female transsexual have the right to visit an OB-GYN before the actual surgery, or only after it?
- Is it fair for an employer to cover Viagra but not birth control pills, since both allow for sexual activity, if in very different ways?
- Speaking of Viagra, exactly how many erections is one worker entitled to in a one-month period?

Although an employer's management of a worker's health care situation seems to devolve to the picayune and the absurd, its inherent intrusiveness is no laughing matter to a worker dealing with depression, HIV, or cancer. Nor is either party happy to engage in financially charged struggles over end-of-life care for a dying family member, or what has proven to be only marginally effective treatments for children with major disabilities, or the rights of a couple like Jim and Jenny to try in vitro fertilization. At $10,000 per cycle and a success rate of roughly 50 percent, the debate over IVF is especially ferocious among large employers with young workforces (Jesitus, 2000). In this instance, determining what an employer should or should not pay for splashes clumsily and loudly into the murkiest waters of medical technology, ethics, and profound human needs. Most employers like Jim's bank are the first to admit that negotiating these types of issues with what is often their most valuable corporate asset—their people—is not a lot of fun. Yet that is precisely what the current system forces them to do. Aside from those in the bank's human resource department who are employed specifically to manage health benefits—and in the process meddle in their fellow employees' personal problems—most employers are not thrilled to be in the health benefits management business.

As a result, employers are split on how they handle the task. As noted, some large employers end up creating and running their own little U.S. health care system. Others are happy to hand the job over to health insurers to do the dirty work for them. And still others choose, if inadvertently, the worst of both worlds by hiring a health insurer to fund and administer their health benefits but then second-guess everything that insurer does. All three options create large, additional infrastructures of imposition in the delivery of health care to employees by third parties who take on the employers' uncomfortable role of saying no. Under all three options, the third parties are caught in the middle between an employer's checking account and its employees' medical needs, forced to figure out what tens of thousands of providers are doing far downstream, and why.

Larger manufacturers like GM have a natural interest in rationalizing the medical delivery system, if only because their corporate cultures expect nothing less of their own operations. A telling example is the intensive involvement by GM in the health care delivered to its employees. The largest private purchaser of medical services in the United States, GM spent $4 billion on health care in 2000 (Carrns, 2001). Because this amounts to more than $1,200 per car (versus $500 for steel for the same car), GM views health care no differently than it views any other production factor: it focuses on the cost and quality of health care services delivered to its employees in the same way it focuses on the cost and quality of its steel, glass, rubber, and other production components (Blumenstein, 1996). As will be discussed in the next chapter, this process is fatally flawed; notwithstanding the Twaddle Echo Factor about managed care, we cannot simultaneously lower costs while improving quality in medicine. But we can at least admire the grandiose ambitions of the effort. GM has deployed productivity teams—precisely the same type of workforce reconfiguration that turned around the entire American auto industry in the late 1980s—to work directly with its health care providers to "reengineer" the way medical services are delivered to GM employees.

"Look at what GM did with Saturn," remarked the president of Genesys Health Care System, a Flint, Michigan, provider system assisted by the GM team. "An entirely new concept of building a car. We decided that health care must also change" (Blumenstein, 1996, p. 1).

Many employers without GM's scale or resources try to accomplish the same reengineering of their health care delivery system on a collective basis.

Many form or join business coalitions designed to micromanage their corner of the U.S. health care system on behalf of their members. These coalitions range from the hundreds of so-called health care purchasing cooperatives around the country (most of which do not do any actual health care purchasing), to the Leapfrog Group, an alliance of large employers that makes occasional, chest-beating pronouncements to the U.S. provider community about what that community is doing wrong and what the group wants fixed. The Leapfrog Group represents companies that provide health benefits to more than 20 million people, spending in the process more than $40 billion per year. In the fall of 2000, the Leapfrog Group announced a plan that will, according to a report in the *Wall Street Journal,* "use their mammoth health-care buying power to press for stringent new safety standards at U.S. hospitals" (Martinez, 2000). The safety standards they are "pressing for" consist of, among other things, hospital purchases of sophisticated, expensive new information technologies that automate their operations, such as electronic drug ordering systems designed to prevent drug-to-drug interactions and other medication errors. Such new information technologies cost several hundreds of thousands of dollars; some of the best cost in excess of $1 million.

But thanks to years of aggressive contracting by large employers and health plans—including, obviously, the Leapfrog Group's own members—these hospitals cannot afford any of the things the group is now pressing for. The same month the group was demanding that providers increase their spending on these and other information technologies, the hospital accreditation group, the Joint Commission for the Accreditation of Healthcare Organizations, was suspending one of its mostly unmet hospital accreditation requirements: passed in the late 1990s, the commission required that hospitals use an approved information system to measure and manage hospital clinical quality. Why the suspension of the requirement? Because such systems, at an average price of $10,000, are too expensive (Lovern, 2000c). This is a crystalline example of how in the multiple, uncoordinated hands of the nation's employers, the U.S. health care system fails, over and over again, to function even remotely like a system. The employers say they want hospitals to invest in quality systems that take years to pay off while in the current year ratcheting down payment rates or failing to intervene when their insurers do so. The employer's chief financial officer wants less expensive health care, the employer's senior vice president of human resources wants higher-quality health care. Who wins? Notwithstanding two decades of rhetoric from the managed care industry, the two do not mix, especially in the short run, and the CFO usually wins.

This is why another pronouncement from the Leapfrog Group is at cross-purposes with the day-to-day purchasing realities of its own members. The group said it plans to "encourage employees to have complicated medical procedures performed at hospitals offering the best survival odds, based in part on the number of procedures a particular hospital performs annually" (Martinez, 2000). Fair enough. Unfortunately, this initiative—if it is actually followed through—will result in driving more patients to higher-cost hospitals—that is, those the group's financial executives least want to take care of their employees. As documented throughout the peer-reviewed medical literature and discussed in a section of the next chapter by the same name, the old adage "You get what you pay for" holds as true in health care as everywhere else in a market economy.

Such employer pronouncements are not anomalies. They are typical of the mixed messages sent to the provider community by large, self-insured companies trying to manage the vast amount of their own money spent by employees like Jim, all of whom have tax-advantaged *dis*incentives to spend it wisely. In this, employers are guilty of the same cost-quality conundrum that the managed care industry has been trying for years to talk its way out of with marketing fluff. Employers want better medical care for less money, a magic formula that does not exist. Able neither to pronounce nor micromanage this fantasy into fruition, they outsource their health benefits to the health insurers, which *do* claim to have the magic formula.

This is not to say that employers have done a great job of figuring out which health insurers offer better quality for the price. After ten years of research, publicity, conferences, and more work, the National Committee for Quality Assurance (NCQA), a group established by employers to measure and compare the performance of HMOs, has yet to drive the HMO selection process for most employers. Despite those ten years of activity, the

NCQA accreditation of health plans, and its much talked-about Healthplan Employer Data and Information Set (HEDIS), has been used by all of 12 percent of U.S. employers. Even more egregiously, those data were made available to only 1 percent of all U.S. employees (Gabel, Hunt, and Hurst, 1998). Through the NCQA, there is a wealth of information regarding which HMOs do a good job of promoting preventive and chronic care, but the CFO's staff at Jim's bank probably did not use it when contracting with PrimeCare. Even if they did, they almost certainly never shared any of that information with Jim. Why? Because PrimeCare may be a crummy HMO that has the special attractiveness to Jim's bank of offering a low premium. The tools employers use to select PPOs is even more dreadful. Even though PPOs cover an estimated 107 million Americans—a far larger market share than the HMOs—only forty-five of the four hundred national PPOs have even bothered seeking accreditation. This is for good reason. Despite the emergence of three PPO accrediting organizations, almost no employers are bothering to check (Lovern, 2001).

One can draw two sorry conclusions from these findings. First, in the grudge match between health care cost and quality that plays out in the executive suites of corporate America, the short-term financial imperative of cost wins. Second, even when quality does actually matter, corporate America is not intent on sharing its plan-selection decisions with its employees. Perhaps this too is because most health insurers' costs and quality levels are directly rather than inversely related, and the last thing an employer wants workers like Jim to know is that based on the best available data it chose a substandard plan for a cheaper price. Some of the twaddle echoing most loudly through the health care system over the past decade involves employers' attempts to talk their way out of this economic reality.

Many of the largest employers have built health care management departments to "walk the talk," staffed with physicians, nurses, outcomes researchers, and medical economists, all engaged in the impossible task of improving the health status of their workforces for contained costs. I have worked with, and have tremendous personal respect for, several dozen corporate medical officers who run these departments. They are talented, dedicated physician-executives, they have made valiant efforts to improve the quality of care delivered to their employees, and many of them have won important victories, if not in the oft-cited management of chronic disease then in critical areas like end-of-life care or detection and management of high-risk pregnancy—two quality improvement initiatives that actually do save money. But collectively, these well-meaning people are fighting a losing battle with their own organizations. They toss out quality initiatives to their contracted health insurers with one hand while the CFO of their organization takes money back with the other. Improving an employed population's health is indeed a job worth doing, if it were actually doable alongside other competing economic pressures.

By the end of the 1990s, the disconnect between employer rhetoric about quality and the cost-related actions employers actually take finally began to show up in disease management and pharmacy costs. Although employers have for years been giving lip service about investing in systems for managing chronic disease among their employees, they have been singularly enraged at increasing expenditures associated with the best weapon we have in the fight against chronic disease: newer, better drugs. This hypocrisy over drug costs may make sense for a health insurer that loses one-fifth of its covered members every year, enjoys no workplace-based economic gains from improved health status of members with major diseases, and thus picks up none of the cost savings associated with a long-run staving off of chronic disease. This same hypocrisy does not make any sense for an employer that gains both in the workplace and over the long term from the discovery of better, albeit more expensive drugs.

The Twaddle Echo Factor surrounding employer-driven health care quality is not limited to plan selection or chronic disease management initiatives. The gap between what employers say they want to do and actually do in practice grows still wider when it comes to measuring the broader corporate benefits associated with health costs. Common sense, not to mention industry punditry, argues that, in numerous instances, the higher medical costs of a self-insured employer may well pay for themselves many times over in reduced absenteeism, higher productivity, and other workplace gains. For example, studies in the late 1980s and early 1990s showed that investments in mental health benefits yield significant gains in workplace productivity while reducing primary care costs. Yet during the same period self-insured employers were shedding mental health benefits as fast as they could, and fully insured employers were shedding them to the degree allowable under state mental health benefit laws.

These parallel trends forced the federal government to step into market in 1996 with its mental health "parity" mandate, a sloppy law that forced all employers, including those self-insured under ERISA, to provide a level of mental health benefits commensurate with their other medical benefits. Because Jim and Jenny live in the "wrong" state, they may not have access to IVF services, but they are free to access mental health counselors, with rich financial coverage, when their frustration and anguish over their medical dilemma metamorphose into full-scale depression.

LIFE IN THE DATA MINES

In defense of the nation's employers, it is difficult if not impossible to measure the broader benefits of investing in a workforce's health status. Doing so would require compiling and analyzing employee experience data in relation to various medical care, operations, and payroll databases—not exactly an easy trick to pull off either technically or legally.

Suppose the human resource professionals—or one of their consultants—at Jim's bank actually could dip into these highly disparate databases and relate the employer's spending inputs on specific drugs, doctors, disease management programs, and other medical care to outputs on employee absenteeism and productivity. This information would be conjured up at great risk to the bank: those medical care databases are political and legal powder kegs. Why? Because a small handful of reprehensible self-insured employers have used access to employee medical records as grounds for terminating health coverage or jobs altogether—choosing to destroy peoples' lives rather than purchase readily available reinsurance—a special coverage that protects self-insured employers against losses on catastrophic employee illnesses. One of the more famous examples of this abuse involved the firing of a Michigan man after his employer looked into his medical claims and saw that he had recently contracted HIV. The man sued his former employer and won a large settlement, in a drama that played out in the national media over several months. Confronted with this and similar isolated, horrifying, and well-publicized episodes, all the Jims and Jennys across the country are receiving health benefits from those they trust least with the details associated with those benefits—their own employers.

This returns us to our central point: an employer-based health care system is stupid. It is the result of a historic accident, it is enshrined in an outdated and unfair part of the tax code, and it simply should not be. The imposition of employers into the health care system introduces a major element of distrust on the part of patients, many of whom may forego needed care, encourage their physicians not to document their medical conditions accurately, or engage in outright fraud to conceal a medical condition from those who could punish them the most for it. The federal government made great strides to remedy some of these abuses by passing the Health Insurance Portability and Accountability Act of 1996 (HIPAA), which made it illegal for an employer to deny health coverage to a new employee with a previously documented medical condition. But HIPAA has created an incentive for employers to redouble their efforts not to hire or promote people with these conditions in the first place: if you hire them, you have to insure them, regardless of what has ailed them in the past.

All of this creates enormous problems for the most well-meaning employers. When Jim's bank wants simply to study the impact of its health benefits decisions on the productivity and health status of its workforce, it is hamstrung by a very real problem of employee perception, one created by a handful of less than well-meaning employers. As a result, most employers, even those with the resources and bandwidth to do so, have failed to integrate medical cost and employment data, further restricting the quality measurement movement and blocking true understanding of the value of innovative medical technologies. My own professional experience ran smack into this problem in the 1990s. Based on the Twaddle Echo Factor popular among self-insured employers at the time, the health information company I worked for, HCIA, acquired and worked hard to expand a business that would pursue exactly these goals: empirical analysis of medical claims and employment data, for the purpose of measuring the real cost-benefits of what employers include in their benefit plans. One of our competitors, Medstat, has been trying to build this same business for more than a decade. And every major employee benefits consulting firm has also tried, with minimal success. A decade later, the state of the art has still not advanced past the same old analysis of medical costs, in a vacuum.

CONTINUITY CONUNDRUM

Under our employer-based private health care system, another important job of the health care system is not getting done and in fact may be getting more undone as time goes by: ensuring continuity of care for people like Jim and Jenny. Because their health insurance is tied to Jim's job, both go away at the same time, leaving these previously insured patients to fend for themselves. The federal government has tried to fix this problem through two important, if piecemeal laws: the Consolidated Omnibus Budget Reconciliation Act of 1983 (COBRA), and HIPAA in 1996. COBRA requires that departing employees have access to continuing coverage, paid for out of their own pockets. Unfortunately, typical COBRA premiums are extremely high, they last for only eighteen months after the employee departs, and they must be paid with aftertax dollars, making them higher still. HIPAA is a better, more progressive law. By making exclusions for pre-existing conditions illegal, HIPAA made it easier for that same employee to sign up for new coverage in the next job, which does away with some of the problems created by COBRA.

But gaps still exist, and this is where the health insurer selection prerogatives of employers hurt employees most. A Kaiser Family Foundation report found that most insured employees have a choice of only one or two health insurers, meaning that when they switch jobs, they usually are forced to switch health insurers as well (Schoen and DesRoches, 2000). This matters less now that most managed care networks have been liquefied to the point of being meaningless, but it still has adverse effects for patients with a disruption in coverage. The same report also found that "those insured but with a recent time uninsured were at high risk of going without needed care and of having problems paying medical bills. This group was two to three times as likely as those with continuous coverage to report access problems." In this, as in so many elements of our hybrid public-private health care system, the United States is the poorest wealthy nation on earth. We spend more money on our health care than any other nation in the world, and yet we spend it incoherently. This incoherence is the very heartbeat of the economic conflict that has always existed between an employer's need to manage the money it spends on health care and its employees' desire to spend as much of that money as possible.

"It's covered," Dave tells Jim, with a matter-of-factness that characterizes a million exchanges between people with good jobs and what they think is good insurance. "Go for it!"

So where do we go from here? Jim's bank may bring purchasing power to the process of health insurer selection. But in so doing, the bank shields Jim and his fellow employees from the costs of their medical decisions, at the expense of restricting their full mobility within the medical system. This may have been a good trade-off when managed care was gaining ground in the early and mid-1990s. But at the tail end of the managed care "revolution," this trade-off of lower price for directed volume is ultimately self-defeating as the MCOs all devolve to open-access models. Health insurers end up offering no meaningful product differentiation, consumers remain locked into an arbitrary set of benefits, and what were once lower prices simply become the new market prices, leading us back to a scarcely altered equilibrium pricing point.

There is a better way to find that same equilibrium point while clearing out all the clutter described in this chapter: give employees pretax dollars that can be spent only on their health care coverage and needs, and give them free and direct access to all health insurers in a market. The insurers would then either have to create real differentiation based on quality or simply compete on price. The result would be a health care market that looks like any other functioning market.

The first step on the road to this marketplace reform is to get employers the hell out of the way. They may give lip service to their role as consumer advocates in navigating the health care system, but because of the inherent economic conflicts—and all the real and perceived potential for abuse—they are highly suspect in that role. Despite the Twaddle Echo Factor generated by talk of the employer as health care consumer advocate, most employers are not especially competent at this anyway, because they assign the management of what may be the most complicated part of U.S. society to human resource departments. Employers are often oblivious to some of the most critical changes in the health care system that directly affect what they purchase for their employees. For example, only 20 percent of those responding to a large survey on state regulation of health plans knew that their states required insurers to spread the cost of small employers with sick employees across a large pool of workers through the use of what are called rating restrictions. Research on this subject found that "only 35 percent of small employers are aware that there are limits on what insurers can charge employers with sick workers compared with employers that have healthier workers. In general, small employers are not knowledgeable about state small-group market reforms passed during the mid-1990s that essentially make it easier for them to obtain and afford coverage" (Fronstin and Helman, 2000, pp. 7–8).

That's the hard evidence; here's an anecdote. In 1997, I sat in on an employee meeting at which a director of the human resource department was explaining the company's recent switch to a new health insurer. A secretary asked, hypothetically, of course, if there would be a problem for people already being "treated for something." The presenter stumbled a bit, clarified that the secretary was asking about preexisting conditions, and then said that because the company wanted to fulfill its obligations to employees, it had decided that preexisting conditions would not be excluded from coverage.

"But doesn't the company have to cover those anyway, with that new law?" the secretary went on, referring to the recent passage of HIPAA, the most significant legislation affecting health benefits in the previous fifteen years.

"I'm not sure," the corporate health benefits director responded. "I'll have to look into that."

I never followed up to see if he got back to her, or if instead he found a reason to have her terminated for whatever hypothetical condition she was suffering from. I do know that, had Jim been in the room, he would have taken a lot of notes and called Jenny with the good news.

The three-pronged reform plan detailed in Chapter Eight of this book is designed specifically to prevent foolish, intrusive conversations like this one from ever having to occur in the first place.

STUCK IN FIFTY CATATONIC STATES

As if a hybrid health care system funded for the most part by both government and the nation's employers did not cause sufficient complexity, confusion, and conflict for society, the federal government thickened the plot by creating—accidentally, of course—two completely different private health care systems. Jim and Jenny are covered by one of those systems; Jim's professional colleague Dave, and his family, are covered by the other. Those PrimeCare insurance cards may look identical, but the medical care that those cards guarantee for two middle-class families in the same community are anything but.

As mentioned in Chapter One, the passage of ERISA back in 1974 to improve the management of pension plans has resulted in the following: 105 million Americans now receive their health coverage through insurers subject to fifty different sets of state regulations, benefit mandates, and oversight procedures, whereas 55 million other Americans receive their coverage through insurers exempt from all state regulations, benefit mandates, and oversight procedures (Wechsler, 2000; Pollitz, Tapay, Hadley, and Specht, 2000). Because of this two-thirds–one-third split, even the largest national health insurers are forced to organize themselves, by default, at the state level.

Small wonder, then, that a decade of consolidations for the purpose of attaining economies of scale and administrative efficiencies (such as Aetna–U.S. Healthcare–NYLCare–Prudential) have fallen apart in execution. Aside from national branding and a few shared administrative services, there is no big national Aetna Health Plan; there are nearly fifty little

Aetna Health Plans, each with its own management staff, regulatory consultants, business processes, provider contracting systems, and claims payment and adjudication circus. These state-level Aetnas all answer to a central governing Aetna, which is responsible for financing, broad policy, the formulation of business strategies, and a handful of information technology initiatives that may or may not be successfully implemented by all the little Aetnas. When Aetna attempted to consolidate three major acquisitions in a few short years, it was really trying to consolidate nearly more than a hundred different state-level health insurers. This explains why it failed to recover from the underwriting cycle with the rest of its industry in the late 1990s and why it missed profit targets in 2000, if not why it was so roundly punished by the same Wall Street that actively encouraged all those acquisitions. Given the problems that inevitably arise when *any* large businesses consolidate, we should not ask why the Aetna experience turned out to be such a financial and operational disaster; rather, we should marvel that it did not turn out even worse.

Operating any state-level health insurer is made especially complex by the permanent presence of the two-thirds–one-third split of the commercially insured population created by ERISA. Most state-level insurers *provide* insurance coverage to employees in fully insured plans subject to state regulations (for example, Dave's plan), while simultaneously *administering* insurance coverage for employees in self-insured plans exempt from those regulations (for example, Jim's plan). The result of the great divide created by ERISA? Workers like Dave and Jim in the same industry who receive the same cash compensation—and who may actually live and work next door to each other and carry what looks like the same health insurance card—are legally guaranteed very different levels of health coverage. Dave and his family may have rich mental health benefits, direct access to specialists, a guaranteed three-day stay for a certain surgery, and the right to sue PrimeCare for a botched medical decision. Though also "covered by" PrimeCare, Jim and his family get none of these things. Some of the people working the information telephones for PrimeCare cannot even figure out the difference.

There is, however, one very important difference between the two kinds of coverage managed by PrimeCare: Jim's bank is paying lower premiums.

Research has shown that exemption from state-based mandates translates into consistently lower premiums. Consumer advocates use this as proof that, left to their own devices, employers would skimp on important coverage and therefore should be forced by mandate to provide more. The other, less obvious reason premiums for Jim's self-insured bank are lower is the cost of compliance with state-based regulation in and of itself, an expense PrimeCare by necessity passes along to Dave's employer. This is our entry point into the vicious cycle created by ERISA, as employers and states play a game of chicken over benefit mandates and their associated costs. The desire of employers with fully insured health plans to pay for less coverage inspires the host state to adopt more mandates; the added costs for those mandates in turn compel more and more employers to seek ERISA exemption to free themselves from *all* state mandates. Paradoxically, each time a state adds a new mandate, it potentially jeopardizes an ever greater number of employees from receiving, literally, the benefits of that very mandate, along with all mandates they currently receive from previous legislative years.

How boneheaded is the growing proliferation of state laws meant to regulate what has consolidated into a mostly national enterprise? Consider the following:

- Thirteen states currently mandate that health insurers either offer or cover some level of infertility treatments (Jesitus, 2000).

- Fourteen states have mental health parity laws that go beyond current federal requirements (Buck, Teich, Umland, and Stein, 1999).

- Forty-three states mandate coverage for services in any hospital emergency room of the patient's choosing, regardless of the true nature of the emergency (Blue Cross and Blue Shield Association, 2000).

- Six states require insurers that cover other prescriptions to include contraceptives ("Federal Agency States . . .," 2000).

- Eight states require coverage for hospice care (Blue Cross and Blue Shield Association, 2000).

- One state allows patients to sue their health insurer for malpractice.

And there is little overlap among states for these benefits. If you live in one state, you are free to start a family at will but not suffer a nervous breakdown; if you live in another, you can go to any emergency room for antibiotics for the flu but cannot sue your health insurer when they kick your husband out of the same hospital while he is suffering from a major postsurgical infection that eventually kills him. Why do some insured Americans have certain medical rights that are seemingly frivolous, whereas others do not have rights that seem outright critical? The answer to this question, like so many answers in health care, is no more rational or intelligible to the average citizen than "just because."

Other problems arise from this fifty-state archipelago of health insurance regulation. The haphazard adoption of state-specific regulations for health plans, originally designed to protect patients from fraud, hamper the widespread adoption of information technologies that would, ironically, greatly improve patient access to care. Notwithstanding the ambitions and representations of dozens of health care Internet entrepreneurs, Web-based processing of medical claims will never occur in several states that still have "quill-and-pen" laws requiring that various medical claims forms be submitted on paper (Havighurst, 2000). Telemedicine services cannot be delivered in several other states, thanks to archaic state reimbursement rules that require physical contact between physician and patient, even though "many consultations could be done effectively over the Internet" (Bentivoglio, 2000, p. 76). Thinking about these and numerous other antiquated state laws regulating health insurance begs the most obvious question: Are fifty different statehouses, with their myriad other legislative agendas, up to the task of regulating an industry as technology-driven, volatile, and complicated as medical care?

The arbitrary state versus federal bifurcation of health plan regulation, played out state by state by state—and all the extra administrative costs, inefficiency, and Chaos Factor they generate—is not only stupid but also completely futile. Forget whatever is actually included in a health plan, and whatever the fine print of each health plan contract says. In fact, American consumers and their lawyers have unambiguous expectations about health insurance coverage that transcends both contract law and the caprices of state regulation. The very idea of benefit plan design itself flies in the face of health care's *real* regulatory system: medical malpractice law. Regardless of what Jim agreed to when he signed up for PrimeCare during his employer's open enrollment period, if Jenny grows seriously ill six months later, the two will demand state-of-the-art medical treatment and they will sue to get it. When confronted with a serious disease and the costs required to treat it, a patient believes one thing: *I have insurance, the premium comes out of my paycheck every week, and this entitles me to whatever medical services are currently available and my doctor thinks are medically necessary.* Jenny (or more accurately, her attorney) also knows that if her doctor were to withhold these services, he or she would be committing medical malpractice; if PrimeCare withholds payment, it is compelling de facto medical malpractice. And *the* cornerstone of medical malpractice law, since 1975, has been the doctrine that there exists across the United States a national standard of care.

Although enormous variations in care exist around the country, the courts hold physicians to a clinical standard that is fully a U.S.–based standard. This standard is determined by medical literature, propagated through training programs and continuing medical education, and confirmed by expert witnesses drawn from any state that Jenny's lawyer chooses for the legal action at hand. This standard is reinforced further by the ultimate sources of most disease-specific medical information for people like Jim and Jenny—namely, the national broadcast, print, and Internet media. Yes, the nationalization of medical care standards operates in a separate sphere of law, but that sphere nonetheless governs physician and patient expectations of what health insurance is supposed to cover. The crazy quilt of state laws covering what health insurance has to pay for is a futile, incomprehensibly redundant effort by state lawmakers to catch up with and encompass those standards. This crazy quilt grows ever more multicolored as local physician community leaders in conjunction with local consumer advocates agitate state legislatures for more mandates.

The obvious fix for this is the shifting of all legislated benefits mandates to the federal level. Such a shift would be consistent with legal doctrine, consumer values, the medical educational role of the national media, consumer and patient activity on the Internet, and common sense. Why not make one law—or no law—instead of thirteen, or sixteen, or twenty-four? It would certainly make running a national health insurer like Aetna much easier, and thus much less expensive. It would also be consistent with recent mandates passed by the federal government that guarantee maternity stays, mental health parity, and health coverage portability—not to mention the national patient's bill of rights, which, as of this writing, is wending its way through a divided Congress. Such federal laws show up through obvious, historic legislative acts like HIPAA, which allow employees to switch jobs and health insurers without risking exclusions for preexisting conditions. They also emerge from less obvious, but equally enforceable federal sources. In 2000, the Equal Employment Opportunity Commission mandated that employers cannot exclude contraceptives from their health benefits plans when they cover other preventive treatments ("Federal Agency States . . ., 2000). In practice, this means that both Jim and Dave's plan—if they cover prescriptions—have to cover birth control pills. Jim's skimpier plan may swallow the cost of the birth control pills; already overburdened by state mandates for things like IVF, Dave's plan may respond by dropping prescription coverage altogether. Stranger ironies occur daily in the tumult of our twin private health insurance systems.

TOWARD A NEW FEDERALISM?

HIPAA was landmark legislation not only because it belatedly guaranteed protection to job-switching employees but also because it signaled a new federalism. "Before HIPAA," writes Karen Pollitz in *Health Affairs*, "health care consumers had dramatically different rights, depending on where they lived or worked and the type of coverage they had or sought" (Pollitz, Tapay, Hadley, and Specht, 2000, p. 8). But all health care reforms proceed in a two-steps-forward-one-step-back pattern. Protections under HIPAA default back to state-based regulation, and "federal enforcement is triggered only when states fail to substantially enforce HIPAA" (p. 9).

Even when clear federal legislative guidance exists, the courts themselves can, operating under their own bizarre ad hoc logic, send health care regulatory processes back to states ill-equipped to administer them. The decision in *Buckman* v. *Plaintiffs' Legal Committee* regarding the liability of medical device manufacturers does not bode well for this fledgling new federalism. Whereas a U.S. District Court in Philadelphia threw out a state court ruling that federal regulation of medical devices preempts state suits, the U.S. Court for the Third Circuit in Philadelphia reversed the ruling. As one observer noted, "It would be quite problematic having state juries decide if federal agencies were misled." But in matters of health care regulation, the Inertia Factor tends to overrule common sense, and inertia will always push important matters back to the states.

WHO BENEFITS FROM THE PROLIFERATION OF BENEFIT PLANS?

The proliferation of arbitrary state-based benefit mandate laws, antifederalist court rulings, and state-by-state regulation of health insurers operating across the country works in favor of two very important intertwined constituencies: the five thousand state insurance bureaucrats who preside over this mess, and the fifty thousand health insurance brokers in bed with them. The brokers, agents, and consultants who tweak and peddle health insurance plans to employers collect commissions ranging from 3 percent to as much as 20 percent of the total cost of those plans (Robertson, 1999). This is an enormous chunk of money, earmarked for medical care, siphoned off by middlemen who add only dubious value to the health care system. If Prime-Care and Dave's bank were not busy coping with and paying all these people out of the company's health care budget, they would probably have more than enough money to pay for the prescription coverage it dropped.

When confronted with this often overlooked leeching off the status quo—this exploitation of the Inertia Factor in health care—health insurance brokers claim that they "add value to employee benefits by helping their clients wade through complicated policies" (Robertson, 1999). These "value-added" services generally involve helping employers create such complicated policies in the first place. Such policies combine whatever benefit mandate the broker's friends in the state legislature happened to pass the previous year, combined with whatever else the broker can talk employers into adding to or taking out of the benefit plan. And I almost forgot: the brokers also do a lot of faxing of health plan enrollment forms to new employees, presumably because the health plans haven't figured out how to use fax machines yet.

The miracle of incomprehensibility that is the typical health benefits policy is an enormous convenience for brokers. Multiplied across thousands of employers and fifty states, the seemingly infinite variations on this miracle provide a simple, credible cover story for what the brokers are really doing: shadow taxing more than $300 billion per year in employer-provided health benefits. This cover story is far more palatable than the truth: brokers are a well-organized business cartel that controls the health insurance distribution channel (Robertson, 1999; Sells, 2000). One major health plan, Wellpoint, spends nearly $300 million on brokers each year, representing 4.3 percent of $6.5 billion in revenues (Robertson, 1999). Most health insurers like Wellpoint receive between 80 and 100 percent of their business through brokers; only one (PacifiCare) has ever had the fortitude to neutralize the brokers' market power and market itself directly to beneficiaries, cutting the brokers out of the middle. Based on what happens to premium rates every year, health care is crying out to fix this problem and eliminate this waste, the same way rises in auto insurance premiums set the stage for direct marketing by insurers like GEICO.

If you think the Internet will change all of this, think again. In 2000, PacifiCare announced that it would offer its HMO plan directly to small employers over the Internet if they chose to sign up on-line, thus minimizing the brokers' administrative role. This directly marketed product carries a highly illustrative discount of 10 percent to 12 percent off prices charged through the traditional broker channel.

"PacifiCare will feel a backlash like never before," one insurance broker told a reporter who asked about the move. "Every agent I know will go out of their way not to write PacifiCare business, and do everything they can to move it."

When de facto collusion does not work to the benefit of brokers, then lobbying and the Inertia Factor do. Even if brokers and their able faxing of enrollment forms *did* add sufficient value to the health care system to justify their extraction of 4 percent of everything employers spend on health care, they are in no hurry to make this easier via the Web. Despite several years of effort and hundreds of millions of burned venture capital dollars, you still cannot purchase health insurance over the Internet in most states. For fully insured health plans—the type of plan that a consumer or small business would purchase "retail" from a broker on the open market—all elements of marketing, plan design, and premiums are regulated by state insurance commissions, which are well greased by insurance brokers.

As will be discussed in Chapter Four, much of what is broken in health care stays broken because it benefits a powerful economic interest. Over the years, certain elements have attached themselves to the health care system like a fungus, health insurance brokers being only one of the more obvious examples. Like a literal fungus, these permanent growths thrive on the health care system's essential complexities and slowness to adapt, on the Chaos Factor and Inertia Factor so pervasive in the industry.

The tax code–compelled imposition of the nation's employers into the health care system—many of them subject to a growing proliferation of state regulations, many others dancing away from those regulations but still on the same state-level health-plan dance floor—cripples all meaningful attempts to improve the system. More of the same may benefit a few special interests but will only increase the insult and injury to Jim, Jenny, Dave, their families, their employers, and their providers. More of the same will guarantee still more shadow taxes, higher premiums, less coverage, and ever greater numbers of people in Jim and Dave's communities with *no* health insurance.

CHAPTER 3

The HMO Will
See You Now

I am reviewing a capitation agreement with a major national HMO for a physician friend, Dr. Elaine Chang. The HMO is offering to pay her practice $9 per member per month (PMPM) for all primary care services. Because I shop aggressively for health coverage for my employees, I know that the HMO charges employers in our market an average premium of $134 PMPM, and assume the payment rate in Dr. Chang's contract is a typo.

"They must mean $19 PMPM," I tell her.

"I'm afraid not," she says. "That's the amount they will pay, take it or leave it. And that $9 is supposed to cover pap smears, vaccines, physicals, flu shots, and all other preventive care services. If we actually provided any of those services—the same ones they promote in their brochures to my patients—we'd be losing money on every single one of them."

It has long since passed into conventional wisdom that the fundamental problem with the U.S. health care system is the existence of a third party to pay for services demanded by the first party and provided by the second party. The economics of this arrangement are forever out of whack because the first two parties stand in direct economic conflict with the third. We would be lucky if the problem were that simple. The imposition of the federal government, fifty state governments, and the nation's employers into the system—the real third-party purchasers of most medical services—has compelled the imposition of fourth, fifth, sixth, and any number of seventh and eighth parties. Respectively, this daisy chain of distinct economic interests consists of health insurance brokers and consultants, national health insurers, state-level operating units of the national health insurers, outsourced vendors of specialty medical services, and countless corporate organizations of providers created specifically to contract with the fourth, fifth, sixth, and seventh parties. By the time a patient covered by that national HMO gets to see Dr. Chang, he may have passed through as many as ten tollgates along the way. Small wonder that in many managed care contracts I have reviewed for other friends and colleagues, a dollar spent on health insurance yields less than a dime for the primary care physician expected to take care of a patient's every basic medical need.

Most of these tollgates are part of the colossus of infrastructure, confusion, and lousy public image known, collectively, as *managed care*. Managed care is an attempt to use market forces to correct the fundamental economic problems that originated within and have since been exacerbated by health care's essential market failures. Under fee-for-service medicine, well-insured patients, many facing the most profound crises of their lives, make unlimited demands on well-paid but poorly organized producers like Dr. Chang and her colleagues. Until contracts like the one I was reviewing came along, neither the patient nor Dr. Chang had any real economic accountability for their decisions. Having been raised with and acculturated through decades of generous insurance coverage, both the patient and Dr. Chang expect the ultimate third party—the employer and government purchaser—to pay for whatever Dr. Chang orders, without questioning the need, price, or outcome. When the third party and all its toll-taking surrogates do not want to pay for what she orders, the patient, Dr. Chang, or their own third-party advocates resort to legislative and legal pressure to defend the order. This is a market-based system?

It is the unhappy job of the nation's managed care organizations (MCOs) to fix this badly broken machine. The fifth, sixth, seventh, and eighth parties that fall under the rubric of managed care—constituting an unintelligible taxonomy of acronyms—attempt to do so by beating on the health care machine; in the process, they accomplish little more than breaking it down even further. The typical MCO is really a Byzantine agglomeration of national, regional, and state-level organizations and cross-contracts. Dr. Chang, who is singularly responsible for the health status of people covered by that MCO, has been reduced to a marginalized figure in one little corner of Byzantium.

Once upon a time, government and employers were fully convinced that the typical MCO could and would simultaneously figure out how to

- Negotiate competitive prices with employers
- Appeal to the employees of their employer-customers
- Appeal to consumers purchasing coverage on their own
- Enroll employees and consumers who decide to become members
- Arrange for every aspect of medical care with tens of thousands of Dr. Changs
- Augment care through arrangements with thousands of institutional providers
- Educate enrolled members about what medical care they really need
- Communicate to all the Dr. Changs how they want them to deliver that medical care
- Block access to that same care if they decide it is not necessary for a member who actually wants it or any Dr. Chang who actually wants to provide it
- Sort through all the paperwork associated with whatever care they *do* decide they will pay for
- Review the same paperwork for potential fraud by all those Dr. Changs and institutional providers
- Stop payment for care that is necessary but results from any kind of workers' compensation, disability, or other event that may have necessitated it
- Write checks for both patients and providers when all other means of not writing them are exhausted
- Analyze the outcomes associated with the care that they do pay for

- Assess thousands of new medical technologies that affect everything they pay for
- Comply with myriad state and federal laws regulating that care
- Build nifty Internet sites
- And, finally, figure out how to make money in the process

Pity the poor MCOs. They are simultaneously pursuing dozens of incredibly complex financial, operational, and marketing goals, many of which are in direct conflict with each other. Unfortunately for doctors like Elaine Chang, providers and their patients end up bearing the brunt of these conflicts.

DIAGNOSIS: ORGANIZATIONAL MULTIPLE PERSONALITY DISORDER

The essential conundrum at the heart of today's MCO is nobody's fault; it stems from a kind of organizational multiple personality disorder created by the impossible role foisted on the MCO by health care purchasers. Out of the long list of business processes involved in managing care, an obvious multiple-choice question emerges: What *is* today's MCO? (a) an insurance company, (b) a provider of actual medical services, (c) a complex transaction processing business, (d) a contract purchasing company, (e) a health services research firm, (f) a data analysis and informatics company, (g) a consumer marketing organization, (h) all of the above. The correct answer is all of the above—the worst possible answer for any business. The only way organizations survive and thrive over the long term is through focus, discipline, and an unambiguousness of purpose. A long list of great American businesses like Federal Express, Sun Microsystems, Home Depot, EDS, Merck, Coca-Cola, Disney, Wal-Mart, Playboy Enterprises, and Patagonia all share one trait: they are single-minded in their ambitions, competencies, and values. By contrast, those like GM, RJR Nabisco, and AT&T, which diversify beyond what they really know and do, always eventually divest.

This simple fact of business life explains why the only MCOs that have really succeeded over time are those that reflect exactly the same qualities of a Federal Express or Patagonia. Kaiser Foundation Health Plan and Group Health of Puget Sound are, compared with the nation's other MCOs, highly stable, focused, and well-defined in their markets. Both are, for the most part, the simplest of HMO models. And as interestingly, both are not-for-profit, and thus economically freer than for-profit MCOs to pursue the privatized public health goals that are, in essence, the real meaning of the phrase *managed care*. The rest of the nation's large MCOs are forever choking on their own sprawl, a sprawl made worse by their ongoing compulsion to acquire, reorganize, and divest each other. They are the victims of the economic and cultural contradictions that arise when one tries to make money by managing care. And they pass along that victimization to patients and doctors like Elaine Chang when these contradictions catch up with them.

Before deconstructing the abject waste of money and energy that defines most of the modern managed care industry, let's review how we let ourselves get this far down a dead-end road. And what a rocky dead-end road it has been. Contrary to popular belief, the modern managed care industry emerged not as a cheaper alternative to indemnity insurance in the late 1980s, but as a left-wing social movement in the early 1970s—an idealized and completely unrealistic alternative to commercial insurance. The typical indemnity health insurance plan back in the 1970s had the same deductibles as today: generally $200 to $500 per year. In 1970, this was a substantial sum of money for the average American family. It left that family accountable for managing a much larger portion of its own medical care than the same deductible does today.

The progressive alternative represented by the vintage 1970s HMO was the result of the strangest possible political bedfellows: retired Vietnam War planners, perhaps contrite over the disaster of geopolitical history they helped exacerbate in Southeast Asia, combined forces with left-wing public health advocates. Together, they engineered a new kind of health insurance organization that owned or controlled its own doctors and hospitals, required *no* deductibles (called first-dollar coverage), emphasized preventive and wellness care, and offered an unusually generous and easy-to-access prescription drug benefit. In a political compromise to counter the left-wing push for nationalized medicine along these same lines, President Nixon sanctioned their creation, signing the HMO Act of 1973, and paving the way for the modern-day MCO. According to colleagues who were involved in those first MCOs (Dr. Chang and I were in elementary school at the time), they were zealous, politically progressive, not-for-profit organizations; their meetings were equal parts political rally, financial planning, and folk music hootenanny. They were an attempt to build an idealized system of socialized medicine—based on some of the more noble if financially unsustainable principles of public health—inside the current system. Their biggest political enemy was not, interestingly enough, the traditional health insurance industry. According to Starr (1982), it was the well-organized, well-funded physician community that, with great prescience, saw the collectivization of contracting under the MCOs as a threat to its financial self-determination. Somehow, the physician lobby sensed—all the way back in 1973—that the collectivization of its services under the first MCOs would one day produce a contract like the one on Dr. Chang's desk today.

For obvious reasons, most of those early MCOs failed, only to be resurrected and repackaged during the health care cost crisis of the middle and late 1980s. As their champions grew up and joined corporate America, the public health premise at the philosophical heart of those early MCOs also got a classic 1980s makeover. Suddenly, the concepts of first-dollar coverage, prevention, and richer drug benefits were fully consistent with the corporate buzzword of the 1980s: they were cost-effective. Nobody had any data to prove this; everybody just assumed it was true. The argument sounded right, and it appealed to two quintessentially American ideals: getting something for nothing, and relying on market forces to figure out how.

The cost-effectiveness premise never worked, a concept we will explore momentarily. For now, the inevitability of that failure explains why, within a decade, managed care went from market-driven panacea for what ails the U.S. health care system to profit-obsessed pariah for everything that is wrong with the U.S. health care system. In the process, the MCOs and their executives were crucified on the cross of public opinion. The media flogged them with anecdotes, the politicians piled on with predictable demagogic ferocity, Hollywood did its characteristic pandering to the public mood du jour, and the lawyers lined up to strip their financial carcasses. The general incomprehensibility of how MCOs actually operate—combined with a few, well-publicized acts of abuse of vulnerable patients—generated a variety of calls for legislative reforms and a raft of class-action lawsuits. The general thrust of those lawsuits was particularly revealing. The commercial MCOs named in the suits were vilified for their failure to announce to the world that managing care, as they practice it, means managing costs.

Go figure. Since the late 1980s, these organizations have been selling a cheaper brand of health insurance and then trying to deliver it on the cheap. Their feel-good TV ads assure Dr. Chang's patients that "our doctors care about you and your family," but the harsh reality of commercial managed care is that Dr. Chang is one of thousands of independent contractors that the MCOs do not trust with "the boss's" money and thus reward financially to care about their bottom line. All the American consumers named as plaintiffs in those legal actions, once they can be contacted and informed of their injuries, are the millions of customers who chose, either directly or through options presented by their employers, low-cost health insurance, only to discover that they were purchasing what turned out to be, lo and behold, low-cost health insurance. The MCOs failed to explain what every American kid learns when she buys her first cheap, imitation chocolate bar: the expensive stuff is better.

Indeed. But time and epidemiology catch up with all of us, and the MCOs are no exception. As healthy people grow older, they eventually get sick. This is exactly what happened to the millions of Americans covered by MCOs as the managed care industry matured. Between the late 1980s and the late 1990s, MCOs carved out a large share of the U.S. health insurance market by focusing their marketing efforts on young, healthy people. The one exception to this proves the rule. The MCOs quickly ramped up their managed care offerings for the elderly on Medicare, and almost as quickly ramped them back down when it turned out—surprise!—that elderly people actually get sick quite often, or at least like to go to the doctor a lot. The MCOs grew to cover a majority of privately insured Americans in less than a decade because they offered a lower-price, cost-constraining alternative to the unlimited choices and access to Dr. Chang offered by traditional health insurers and the Medicare program. It was inevitable that these same organizations, including the HMO whose contract I reviewed for Dr. Chang, would come under political, popular, media, and legal attack for seeking to constrain costs. How they do so is a classic lesson in caveat emptor: when people sign up in December for the lowest-price health coverage offered by their employer or Medicare, they are in for a surprise in June should they actually need care. The likelihood of this increases for Dr. Chang's patients, of course, if she accepts that contract and "forgets" to provide those preventive services.

If there is any culpability for the national HMO in all of this, it is the essential bait-and-switch it is pulling on Dr. Chang's patients who sign up in December. Despite those lower premiums, that HMO actually offers richer benefits than traditional coverage; the trick is the obstacles it creates for patients trying to access them. Cheaper insurance premiums for richer guaranteed benefits create one overriding imperative for the commercial HMO: it has every incentive to reduce costs, put the financial screws to Dr. Chang, contract with the cheapest hospitals in town, and micromanage every aspect of their clinical behavior. Enter stage right, the class-action lawyers who, like Louie in the film *Casablanca*, are shocked, shocked, to find economic motives impinging on professional behavior!

The typical MCO's marketing puffery about providing "quality" health care is exactly that. In a market economy, where economics will always drive excellence, higher quality *anything* translates into higher prices: better cars, snappier hotel service, a warmer coat, network versus premium cable television programming—and unfettered access by insured people to the best medicine. The hysteria among MCOs over the past few years over their rapidly increasing pharmacy costs is the most crystalline example of the central paradox of managed care. The MCOs have always provided more comprehensive drug benefits—this is how they lured millions of Medicare beneficiaries to their plans—based on the self-evident principle that better drugs, when used appropriately, translate into better management of disease. After a decade of better drug benefits and MCO-driven disease-management strategies, the MCOs suddenly started chafing against the direct costs associated with exactly what they were offering the market. Why?

Because the reality of more generous prescription benefits was pure marketing all along, more good stuff for less money.

Better doctors, like better drugs, also cost more. And they cost more not only directly but also indirectly. A little noticed but powerful study published in *JAMA* found a direct relationship between physician scores on board exams and the intensity of resources they ordered for their patients. According to the study, "Licensing examination scores are significant predictors of consultation, prescribing, and mammography screening rates in initial primary care practice" (Tamblyn and others, 1998, p. 989). This illustrates a fairly straightforward piece of common sense: if Dr. Chang is a smarter doctor, she will be more cognizant of a greater variety of clinical problems potentially affecting her patients and thus will order more diagnostic tests to rule them out. These patterns of "high utilization" are precisely what the MCOs focus on most intensively when recontracting with physicians like Dr. Chang. They "ding" them for delivering more care; at the extreme, they kick them out of their networks altogether if they do not adapt.

Though it is rarely mentioned in polite company, the MCOs do *not* seek to promote and pay for better doctors and medicines. Instead, they promote and pay for cheaper doctors and medicines, and hope for the same outcome. To this end, the MCOs have built enormous infrastructures designed to do one thing: just say no. Most large MCOs maintain their own internal army of well-meaning physician-executives, biostatisticians, economists, data analysts, and public health experts. But these are not the people running the organizations. The chief medical officers who direct these armies use the data to decide what medical services to pay for, which to promote aggressively to members, and which to deny. They are responsible for "how the medical-services portion of the budget should be spent," according to Thomas Bodenheimer and Lawrence Casalino, writing in the *New England Journal of Medicine.* "Final decisions are generally made by the executive officers rather than by the medical directors" (Bodenheimer and Casalino, 1999). Why? Because those officers are themselves in charge of even larger internal armies of accountants, financial managers, utilization reviewers, and claims auditors; *these* are the people running the MCOs.

Using numbers crunched by the chief medical officer's army, yet a third army—the marketing and sales people—produces white papers and PowerPoint presentations galore to show their employer-customers that they add value sufficient to justify the chunk of the health insurance premium dollar they lop off to feed their three armies.

DATA SPEAK LOUDER THAN TV ADS

Time for a reality check. A comprehensive survey of the peer-reviewed medical and health services literature shows *no meaningful improvements in health status, access, or outcomes for people in managed care versus nonmanaged care insurance systems. Often, it shows a decline.* A study in the *Milbank Quarterly* found "little evidence of any consistent difference in clinical quality between FFS [fee-for-service plans] and HMOs . . . we found no conclusive evidence that FFS plans provide either consistently better or consistently worse quality of care than HMOs" (Dudley, Miller, Korenbrot, and Luft, 1998, p. 673). In fact, despite all the managed care rhetoric about improving population health, the most comprehensive evidence shows precisely the opposite: across an entire insured population, managed care actually does more harm than good. A landmark, four-year study comparing the health status of Medicare patients in the traditional program with those in managed care plans found that patients have "worse physical health outcomes in HMOs than in FFS systems" (Ware, 1996, p. 1039). Given the financially onerous terms of Dr. Chang's contract, is this deterioration in health status a surprise?

In the mid-1990s, after a protracted political debate, the second of two Medicaid populations was handed over to an MCO, TennCare in Tennessee, a move that a number of other states quickly followed. One of the supposed goals of the transition (as packaged for state legislators and the media) was to coordinate services, reduce cost, and improve the clinical quality of care delivered to pregnant women and their newborns. Did it work? According to a study in *JAMA*, "Perinatal outcomes did not change among Medicaid births following the transition to TennCare" (Ray, Gigante, Mitchel, and Hickson, 1998, p. 314). One of the arguments for moving the Medicaid population to managed care was based on the managed care industry's pitch that it could right a chronic wrong in the U.S. health care system: barriers to care for the nation's minority populations. But a broader analysis of access to care by minorities five years after the conversion of Medicaid programs to managed care in several states has not borne this out: "Minorities, particularly Hispanics and Asian Americans, were more likely than non-Hispanic whites were to report barriers" under managed care (Phillips, Mayer, and Aday, 2000, p. 65).

A hallmark of managed care, at least according to the MCOs' marketing literature and public relations pronouncements, has always been their supposed ability to diagnosis dread diseases like cancer early. Unfortunately, the evidence does not support this. According to research published in *Medical Care,* early diagnosis of breast cancer was the same for patients in both managed care and nonmanaged care systems. The results do not get any better when it comes to the treatment of breast cancer once diagnosed: "Survival of group-model HMO, nongroup-model HMO, and FFS patients was not significantly different" (Lee-Feldstein, Feldstein, Buchmueller, and Katterhagen, 2000, p. 705). The same study found that what *does* matter is not the type of health insurance a patient has, but the type of provider. "Group-model and nongroup-model HMO patients are similar to FFS-insured patients in stage at diagnosis and survival outcomes," the study noted. "Treatment selection is related to hospital type rather than insurance coverage" (p. 705). This failure is not limited to breast cancer. For the diagnosis and treatment of colon cancer, another major killer that can often be successfully conquered with early detection, the MCOs fare no better. According to a study in the *American Journal of Public Health,* patients with colorectal cancer insured by commercial HMOs actually had *higher* mortality rates than patients with traditional insurance (Roetzheim and others, 2000). So much for the expensive, well-intended cancer prevention efforts of thousands of commercial MCOs.

Their recurring failure to make any difference in clinical quality hits the MCOs on the medical turf they defend most ferociously. A specific clinical example repeated almost mantralike by the medical directors of MCOs is the large percentage of physicians who fail to follow clear and unarguable medication guidelines for treating heart attack patients. Those guidelines state that patients discharged from the hospital following a heart attack should be given both aspirin and beta-blockers, two inexpensive and generally safe treatments. The large share of patients *not* given this basic level of care even made the front page of the *Wall Street Journal.* The story touted United Healthcare's efforts to correct this situation, which it did through the heroic efforts of one highly motivated medical director (Burton, 1998). United Healthcare's success story made the front page of a major publication because it is the managed care exception, not the rule. According to a study of patients across multiple MCOs, published in the *Journal of General Internal Medicine,* "Use of aspirin and beta-blockers was comparable among HMO and FFS patients" (McCormick and others, 1999, p. 73). This failure of the MCOs to effect so basic and indisputable a clinical reform probably explains why a separate study found no difference in outcomes between elderly heart attack patients in managed care versus nonmanaged care settings. The authors of this second study *did* find differences in heart attack treatment, but they were not related to insurance type; the differences were associated with physician status, with younger physicians more likely to follow the treatment guidelines than older ones (Soumerai and others, 1999). Once again, what seems to matter in health care is what kind of doctor takes care of the patient, not who is trying to shove a $9 PMPM primary care contract down her throat.

The failure of MCOs to perform better than unmanaged health insurance systems is almost certainly the result of the special barriers to access that the MCOs create, ironically, in their bungling attempts to rationalize the care delivery process. Like the liberal pharmacy benefits they whine about when their members use them liberally, across the rest of the medical system the MCOs tend to give with one hand and take away with the other. They spend a tremendous amount of money fighting their own efforts, and in the end these efforts cancel each other out. According to a study comparing resource use by patients in managed care versus nonmanaged care systems, published in *Health Services Research,* "few differences are observed in [medical] service use, such as preventive care, hospital use, and surgeries" (Reschovsky, Kemper, and Tu, 2000, p. 219). The same study found that "in total, differences in adjusted service use across the four [different insurance types] range from no detectable effect on many services to a five percentage point difference in the likelihood that the last physician visit was to a specialist" (p. 226). Numerous other studies either confirm this or find that the managed care hand giving more access is overpowered by the managed cost hand taking it away. In terms of overall access to medical care, a study published in the *Archives of Internal Medicine* found that "the managed indemnity system performed most favorably. Point of service and network-model HMO performance equaled the indemnity system on many measures. Staff-model HMOs performed least favorably, with adjusted mean scores that were lowest or statistically equivalent to the lowest score on all 10 scales" (Safran and others, 2000, p. 69).

Another hallmark of managed care is, in theory, the long overdue introduction of continuity and coordination of care in what has always been a fragmented, poorly organized medical community. Once again, however, actual experience shows that managed care as practiced over the years has yielded exactly the opposite. "The reduced patient-physician continuity observed in [managed care] plans is consistent with previously reported data and appears to hold critical implications for both the quality and cost of care," concludes one researcher in *JAMA*. "Organizational access, continuity, and accountability were highest in the FFS system . . . comprehensiveness was lowest in HMOs" (Safran, Tarlov, and Rogers, 1994, p. 1579). This is one of the supreme paradoxes of managed care: the MCOs' often Herculean attempts to make the health care delivery system work better for patients is subverted by the disruptions perpetuated by those very attempts. The MCO may want Dr. Chang to provide those preventive services and higher quality care, but its contracting actions speak louder than its TV ads.

MCO MULTIPLE PERSONALITY DISORDER, DECONSTRUCTED

In an exhaustive, two-part *New England Journal of Medicine* analysis of how MCOs actually operate, Robert Kuttner (1998a, b) explored the origins of managed care's behavioral paradoxes. Managed care mechanisms, he writes, "entail an endless regress of private regulation—multiple and often over-lapping sets of practice guidelines, quality audits, utilization reviews, physician profiling, and at-risk incentive formulas modified by appeals systems and ethical constraints" (1998b). Kuttner's survey of the industry reveals the extent of the Chaos Factor generated by managed care: "There are now literally thousands of sets of clinical-practice guidelines and as many data systems as there are HMOs and other health plans" (1998b).

These thousands of data systems and private sets of guidelines are propagated and presided over by enormous bureaucracies, each with highly duplicative sets of rules—though not predictably duplicative, which would make Dr. Chang's clinical life much easier—that effectively block patient access to her care. This observation goes a long way in explaining Safran's earlier finding that "HMO patients rate their telephone and appointment access less favorably than FFS patients" (Safran, Tarlov, and Rogers, 1994). It also explains why, according to a separate study in *Health Services Research,* "Enrollees in more managed products are less likely to cite financial barriers to care but are more likely to perceive problems in provider access, convenience, and organizational factors" (Reschovsky, Kemper, and Tu, 2000). Such findings confirm the cynicism of the industry's worst critics: managing care really means managing away patient's access to care. Once again, the MCO gives with one hand, and takes away with the other.

These forces are at the very heart of the MCO's corporate culture of just saying no. How they actually work was revealed in damning testimony given to Congress by Linda Peeno, an idealistic physician turned managed care medical director. Dr. Peeno tells a compelling story about how economic and organizational pressures pervading her MCO forced her always to look for a way "to say 'no.' If I cannot pronounce it medically unnecessary, then I have to find a different way to interpret our medical guidelines or the contract language in order to deny the request. Though factors like budgets, networks, and contracts make critical differences," she writes, "once a plan is up and running, the quickest way to a good bottom line is to limit and deny services. And the industry message was clear: that is the medical director's job" (Peeno, 1998).

In a deeply disturbing article entitled "What Is the Value of Voice?" Dr. Peeno describes her epiphany as an MCO medical director. A covered member who had lost her voice to a rare condition required an expensive piece of technology that would restore it, and allow her to speak, work, and function. Dr. Peeno's peers at the MCO browbeat her, insisting that she not authorize payment for the device. Nonetheless, her conscience prevailed. "When I approved the request," she reports, "I got a call from my physician supervisor, angrily telling me that we did not pay for 'creature comforts.' Under such industry-wide unspoken guidelines, no doubt, a voice would be considered a creature comfort" (Peeno, 1998).

Dr. Peeno's story is a disturbing little anecdote from a nationwide chorus of disturbing little anecdotes. Hers is the experience of thousands of other once-idealistic physicians and health administrators trapped in a system that makes sense only when we step back and remember that it was conceived, in part, by a handful of technocrats who directed American involvement in the Vietnam War. With apologies to Dr. Alain Enthoven, whom I know personally and respect tremendously, it is important to review what he and his colleagues originally tried to do in the early 1970s. After failing to engineer a military "solution" to communist encroachment in Southeast Asia, they attempted to engineer a commercial solution to cost inflation in fee-for-service medicine. The hubris embodied in both of these efforts—and American society's initial embrace of the second one—speaks volumes about how we got this far down the dead-end road of managed care. As a culture, we have an abiding faith that enough technology, planning, data, and perseverance will conquer any problem. In the 1960s, this faith got us to the moon, one of our great national triumphs. This same faith also embroiled us in an ugly civil war we could not win, with or without full public support. Vietnam remains one of our nation's greatest sources of pain, a wellspring of anguish for those who served and suffered, for those who protested, and for those looking back who were not old enough at the time to do either.

Managed care has inspired a less acute version of the same anguish across the country. The substantive differences between these two very different national experiences, the moon shot and Vietnam, explain why managed care's reengineering of health care is not working. Going to the moon involves physics, math, engineering, athleticism, meteorology, and luck; winning a civil war on behalf of an ambivalent and divided "ally" involves reengineering human conflicts and historic realities. Fixing the U.S. health care system is analogous to the second effort, not the first. Like the jungles and cities of Vietnam, the U.S. health care system is a messy, scary, confusing, unpredictable place, full of tangled alliances and deep mistrust. In designing the chaos of administrative microprocess that is the modern MCO, Vietnam's apostate war planners blew it a second time. As stated in Chapter One, they replaced the chronic disorganization of American medicine with acute overorganization. As Dr. Ronald Glasser observes, "Cadres of systems managers, some of whom had planned the failed technowar in Vietnam, brought forth new corporate structures meant to introduce market forces into the industry and named by the several acronyms for preferred or managed medicine" (Glasser, 1998, p. 36). Only those with hubris enough to believe that military technology can overcome historic shifts in geopolitical power could also believe that we can "plan" our way out of the simplest facts of life. As people get older and sicker, they will consume more health care, not less, and they will not tolerate the de facto rationing of medicine that is the result of all managed care planning, however well intentioned. (Interestingly, this same hubris inspired the technocratic planning monstrosity at the core of the Clinton Health Care Reform Plan of 1994, a fact so glaring that even the most casual observer seemed able to identify it as such.)

The MCOs are losing their war against medical costs for many of the same reasons we lost the war in Vietnam, and for all the reasons we as a nation rejected the Clinton plan: in health care, we can neither plan, nor systematize, nor "technologize" our way out of the inevitable. If there is one overriding message from all the clinical research cited earlier, it is this: managed care has failed to attain the public health goals central to its own conflicted missions. This is no one's fault; it is simply a fact of life. The profit motives and corporate management of commercial MCOs, focused as they are on quarterly financial targets, clash with the ideals of wellness, prevention, early diagnosis, and real disease management. In this, the MCO cul-

66

ture of just saying no reveals its most fundamental contradiction: managed care is an attempt to commercialize public health, an economically unsustainable proposition. How did we get so turned around on this? Once again, a look back at the history of managed care is highly instructive.

When the commercial MCOs were first marketing themselves to corporations in the late 1980s, they did so on the presumption that they would be, as stated earlier, cost-effective. (The current version of this same buzzword is ROI, short for *return on investment,* which is really just cost-effectiveness retooled for the 401k crowd.) The notion that richer health care benefits are actually cost-effective—or that they "have a positive ROI"—may sell well to corporate executives who value their own personal wellness and prevention, but they do not stand up to the facts. Higher quality care is *not* cost-effective; wellness and prevention do *not* save money; trying to make an insured population healthier is actually more expensive than letting it flounder, especially in the short run. This is the central finding of the landmark work on the subject, *Is Prevention Better Than the Cure?* written by Louise Russell of the Brookings Institute. Though Russell published her work in 1986, a few short years before MCOs sank their teeth into the employer health care dollar, we can only assume that few of those corporate managers hearing the MCO's cost-effectiveness pitches bothered to read it.

The dreary realities of population health cost accounting go a long way in explaining the failure of managed care to deliver on its more noble promise—and why the culture of just saying no always wins out over the culture of just making them healthier. These realities can be summed up in one chilling example: treating a handful of runaway breast cancer cases is a lot cheaper than providing mammograms for hundreds of thousands of healthy women. As compassionate people, horrified by the very thought of breast cancer, we shrink from so cruel a calculus; as effective marketers, so do the MCOs. In collective denial of this reality since they first started marketing to employers, they spend enormous amounts of time and energy preaching the value of prevention, wellness, early diagnosis, and "quality" out of one side of their mouths—while screaming at hospitals, drug companies, and doctors like Elaine Chang about costs out of the other. This explains why the typical MCO goes to great lengths to promote the immunization of newborns in its population, while actually reimbursing physicians for less than the acquisition cost of the vaccines (Grimes, 2000).

Despite the failure of managed care to improve clinical outcomes for those it covers, the public health news in the United States is actually quite good. With the exception of a widespread rise in diabetes incidence, health status for the nation as a whole is improving. Heart disease patients are living longer and better, cancer mortality rates are declining, immunization rates are up, and as a whole our life expectancy continues to expand—all remarkable feats considering how difficult it is to make such gains in a society as affluent and sophisticated as ours. As the clinical research cited earlier makes clear, such improvements, at least for the commercially insured population, are the same regardless of who provides the insurance.

So whom should we credit, if not the MCOs, for all the good news? Although there is no hard evidence to support this, I would argue that these improvements are attributable to several interrelated sources, all of which ultimately flow from the busy research labs and enormous, oft criticized marketing budgets of the nation's drug companies:

- The media, both traditional and Internet-based, and its expanding role in educating consumers and patients about prevention, wellness, and treatment breakthroughs
- Better medicines and other medical technologies, which MCOs generally resist paying for until forced to do so
- The efforts of drug companies to find and market better cures
- The slow-but-steady advent of evidence-based medicine, a data-driven clinical practice phenomenon that originated in Canada, not the United States
- The mushrooming of drug company advertising that most MCOs find so loathsome
- A younger generation of better-trained physicians, who receive almost all of their clinical education after medical residency either directly or indirectly from the drug companies

In direct contrast to the financial accounting of the MCOs, the "outrageous" profitability of the drug companies works in favor of patients, not in favor of MCO shareholders at patients' expense. A glossary moment is in order here. Every time an MCO pays for a vaccine, mammogram, surgery, new drug, or extra visit to Dr. Chang, the cost for that medical service is added to its medical *loss* ratio. Though an imprecise measure, the medical loss ratio is useful for comparative and illustrative purposes; it is defined as the share of the premium dollar spent on actual medical care versus administration, broker commissions, and profits. When investments in population health are viewed through the financial prism of an MCO's medical loss ratio, it is easy to argue that we have won our recent improvements in public health *despite* the efforts of managed care to reduce collective access to medical care.

The MCOs got us so turned around on this issue because they are not speaking for us, their members, and they are certainly not speaking for Dr. Chang. They are speaking for their real customers, the nation's employers. The commercial MCOs know who their bosses are, and they know the dirty work they must do on their behalf. They successfully packaged and sold an untenable, two-sided proposition that has failed—if only because they were able to attain the first part of this proposition for a brief moment in health care history. Employers want lower cost and higher quality; unable to get them both at the same time, they will always default to the former at the expense of the latter. Anyone who thinks otherwise should be in the room when the CFO of a large company is looking at comparative MCO performance data, choosing which MCOs to contract with next year, and figuring out co-premium rates for the company's workers.

The resulting pricing pressure from that CFO puts a double squeeze on the MCOs. They are economically motivated to just say no more often; these efforts then risk alienating the MCO's covered members and driving them to opt out of the plan, thus costing the MCO money in the marketing expense category. In effect, the MCO is forced to make a miserable business decision: Do we trade down medical costs for higher marketing costs? A look at disenrollment data would indicate how for-profit MCOs make their decision. One survey found that "low disenrollment rates are related to nonprofit status of plans. Seven of the ten plans with the highest disenrollment rates were for-profit, while nine of the 10 plans with the lowest disenrollment rates were nonprofit" (Dallek and Swersky, 1997). Unfortunately, because of the utter size and complexity of the health care system—and because of the imposition of the employer into the system in the first place—the economic imperative created by employers and embodied in the MCO culture of just saying no is not contravened by marketplace forces. The same survey found that the MCOs with the greatest turnover in members do not suffer for it financially. Among MCOs with the largest disenrollment rates, the survey found that many "continued to stay in business, and in some cases grew, despite disenrollment rates of over 20 percent" (Dallek and Swersky, 1997). The Chaos and Inertia Factors strike again.

WHO BUYS AN OUNCE OF PREVENTION?

Disenrollment rates as high as 20 percent make any real investment in a covered population's health status a fool's pursuit. Why should that national HMO pay Dr. Chang more to provide cancer screenings, when those screenings will save its competitors cancer treatment costs three, four, or five years down the road? Truly managing care requires a stable population, one in which the MCO can invest real medical resources, measure the results, and reap the financial rewards in the long term, if there are any. This truism, combined with the lower disenrollment rates for the not-for-profit MCOs, leads us to one obvious conclusion: the closest we get to true managed care is nonprofit.

Once again, we return to where we began, to fiercely not-for-profit MCOs like Kaiser and Group Health, the nation's first HMOs, and still the nation's most successful. As Kuttner reports, "In the Pacific Business Group on Health's 1997 rankings, Kaiser remained the top-rated California HMO. And notwithstanding competitive pressures, Kaiser has retained adjusted community rating, at least in California, and does not practice risk selection in its marketing. With relatively low disenrollment rates and half a century of experience, Kaiser has perhaps the most comprehensive patient data

70

base of any health plan, which it uses to promote integrated patient care" (Kuttner, 1998a, p. 1560). In all of these dimensions, what Kaiser does is consistent with the public health goals of real managed care. By the same measures, the aggressive adverse-risk avoidance, highly differential premium rating, and constant enrollment turnover by the for-profit MCOs belies what they really are: health insurance companies in managed care packaging. All marketing twaddle.

This inevitable conclusion about who is really managing care is confirmed by comparisons of medical loss ratios for MCOs by profit status. Not-for-profit plans on average have medical loss ratios of 90 percent, versus the 80 percent for most not-for profit plans, and as little as 60 percent for some of the most ferociously managed MCOs (Kuttner, 1998a). Kaiser's medical-loss ratio percentage is usually in the mid-90s; Group Health's is 92 percent (McCue, 1998). In sharp contrast to what these not-for-profits do for their members, the MCOs that spend as little as 80, 70, or only 60 percent of the premium dollar on medicine are not managing care. Instead, they are managing money, and doing it quite well (*HCIA Guide to the Managed Care Industry*, 1995–1998). So much for the marketing twaddle.

Why doesn't the marketplace sort this out? Because our tax code has embedded employers in the system, who in turn direct most of the commercial health insurance consumer traffic in the marketplace. If we had complete freedom to choose where we spent our premium dollar, we would surely choose a plan that gives us 90 cents of that dollar back in medical care, not 60 cents. The problem, once again, is that most of us do not have that choice. We are beholden to the choices made by our employers—decisions that are influenced by the corporate goal of lower premiums, not higher medical loss ratios.

The real danger of this chronic marketplace distortion is a competitive "race to the bottom" that the for-profit MCOs have initiated on behalf of their employer-customers. Because they spend so much less of the premium dollar on medical care, the commercial MCOs were able to drag Kaiser and Group Health into a bidding war that resulted in significant losses for everybody, the for-profits included, in the late 1990s. The result was financial catastrophe not only for all the MCOs but also for vast numbers of providers on the whipsaw end of the cost-cutting process. Dr. Chang's contract with that major HMO is a clear reflection of this process. The short-sighted, profit-driven commercialization of the entire managed care industry is a serious threat to the original mission of the not-for-profit MCOs. Kuttner says it best, with a bitter rhetorical question: "Has the competitive pressure to cut costs reached a point where socially oriented HMOs embrace practices they once abhorred just to stay in business?" (Kuttner, 1998a, p. 1559).

The very notion of commercial managed care is the most preposterous oxymoron in the panoply of oxymorons that define the U.S. health care system. It is a so-called marketplace solution that serves only to aggravate the original problem, and for one simple reason: there is almost no real marketplace for health care coverage in the United States. The purchaser of health coverage is not its real consumer; indeed, the purchaser usually has goals that conflict with the consumer's goals. As a result, the product is rarely what the consumer really wants. No amount of tinkering, piecemeal legislation, MCO pronouncements, or industry twaddle will change this fundamental disconnect, one that now pervades half the U.S. health care landscape.

The biggest ramification of this disconnect should by now be obvious. With the exception of anomalies like Kaiser and Group Health, managed care practices none of what it preaches. Those practices are propagated throughout the system through contracts like the one confronting Dr. Chang for a large number of her patients. If she behaves the way the contract compels her to, skimping on preventive services to minimize her financial losses, then we can draw but one conclusion: commercial managed care has failed, except perhaps as a middle-class jobs program for all those people inside the MCOs working so hard on all of their ultimately conflicting tasks. Any meaningful reform of the U.S. health care system should focus the bulk of its energy on fixing this disconnect; it should seek, first and last, to rechannel the vast sums of money that most of managed care has been extracting from the system and use that money instead to pay for people's medical care.

YOU GET WHAT YOU PAY FOR

In medicine, progress is expensive. For every new pharmaceutical product that makes it to market, five thousand other promising compounds fail (personal communication, Jeff Truett, spokesperson, Pharmaceutical Research and Manufacturers of America, Jan. 2001). The winner has to pay for all those losers, currently half a billion dollars worth of research and development costs. When we pay $60 for a handful of what look like cheap chemicals, what we are really buying is a piece of one drug company's winning lottery ticket. And although many new drugs will save money in the short run by reducing more expensive interventions like surgeries and hospitalizations (a concept most MCOs have yet to figure out), the long-run economic effect of most new drugs is still more spending. People who would have died without the new drug go on to live longer and consume still more medical resources.

Thanks to breakthroughs in antibiotics and vaccines in the early twentieth century, we had the good fortune as a society of living long enough to discover the patience of heart disease and the inevitability of cancer. Thanks to great progress in the second half of the twentieth century treating heart disease and cancer, we have had the good fortune as a society of living long enough to discover something called Alzheimer's disease. Breakthroughs in imaging and other diagnostic technologies today allow Dr. Chang to diagnose diseases in her patients they did not know they had until too late. Now Dr. Chang and her medical specialist colleagues can treat those diseases earlier and in more patients, ultimately placing still greater economic burdens on society. For Dr. Chang's surgeon colleagues, new technologies broaden the indications for and utilization of entire spheres of surgery that, even if less expensive than cruder versions of the same procedure or palliative care in the short run, also allow people to live longer lives and consume still more health care.

This essential feature of medicine seems to have eluded those who purchase and manage health care. It is the obvious source of mystification and perplexity among those in government and corporate America forever railing against national health care expenditures that grow faster than our gross domestic product. Of course growth in our medical expenses is outstripping growth of our GDP! As a society we are getting ever older, more affluent, more educated, more demanding, and more sensitive to our own health status. This is a sign of social progress; it signifies our collective migration up what psychologist Maslow refers to as our hierarchy of needs. This disproportionate growth of medical spending is also a macroeconomic inevitability, as our food, housing, and transportation needs grow ever easier to meet through production economies of scale that do not exist in medicine, using technologies that do not change as fast as our medical technology does. Such progress is not cheap.

As was shown at length earlier in this chapter, we have tried to talk our way around this problem. The more-for-less marketing promises of the MCOs convinced us that we could simultaneously invest in medical progress while somehow paying less than what that progress costs. Oops. The real culprit is our native idealism and corollary misunderstanding about medical economics, and our resulting willingness to swallow whole—at least for a time—the Orwellian advertising copy spewed out by the MCOs when packaging those economics into a newfangled kind of health insurance plan. As patients, we believe that better medicine lowers costs because it makes us healthier. As professionals, we believe that, like the economies of scale associated with producing food, housing, or transportation, a decade of mergers and acquisitions will produce the same economies in health insurance and medicine. But the utter complexity of the private and public health insurance systems, combined with the Inertia Factor that complexity promulgates, robs us of those economies. And medicine, for all the attempts to corral its delivery into corporations, is and will forever be more local service business than national technology enterprise. All the Twaddle Echo Factor about the human genome project notwithstanding, new medicines are still discovered and tested mostly by hand, and prescribed entirely by hand, by hard-pressed doctors like Elaine Chang. There is no economic leverage in any of this, just economic pressure when we demand more.

The news media, meanwhile, does not sleep. Aware of the changing demographics and obsessions of its audience, the media is increasingly responsible for driving our insatiable appetite for more, better, newer medicines. The daily newspaper, nightly network news, and Web are all filled with a growing torrent of medical research that promotes one idea: faster, more aggressive, more technologically enriched medical treatment works. And it is no accident that most of the national advertising on the network news broadcasts, in publications dedicated to health news, and splashed across (or hiding behind) most health care Internet sites comes from one source: the drug companies.

Consider a front-page article in the *Wall Street Journal,* a story repeated by two of the four major news networks the same day, and featured on several major Internet portals over the days that followed. According to the report, "The rate of heart attack or death alone was reduced by about one-third to 6.3% for aggressive treatment, compared with 9.5% in the conservative group." Further, patients referred quickly for a diagnostic angiogram and possible angioplasty or bypass surgery were "18% less likely to die or suffer a major heart attack or other adverse event than those whose evaluations were stretched out across several days and included an exercise-stress test to determine if an angiogram was necessary" (Winslow and Hensley, 2000, p. B1). As these findings are replicated throughout the health care system by physicians adopting the well-publicized protocols, the cumulative result of reduced mortality for this large patient population will be more heart disease patients living longer, consuming more drugs and hospital days, and eventually getting cancer and Alzheimer's disease. Good news for patients, their loved ones, their doctors, and the drug companies—and terrible news for the actuaries and other bean counters at large companies, MCOs, and the HCFA, all of which will have to bear the added economic burden of these improvements.

An empirically driven compulsion toward more aggressive care, delivered faster and for more patients, is especially powerful when it comes to heart disease, the nation's most prevalent and costly major medical condition. Over the past decade, the U.S. hospital community has been overwhelmed by the added costs stemming from a series of technical breakthroughs in heart surgery involving minimally invasive technology. Balloon angioplasties, originally thought to lower health care costs by reducing the number of bypass surgeries, are having the opposite effect.

Whereas the number of CABGs has remained constant, still more patients are eligible for the less invasive angioplasty alternative, thus increasing the total heart surgery bill for the nation (*HCIA National Inpatient Profile,* 1992–1998; Fuchs, 1999). And as the procedure itself is continually refined and studied by researchers, it is being enhanced with related therapies. The mid-1990s saw the launch of a new class of drugs that inhibited platelet aggregation around the intravascular site of the angioplasty; these drugs added several thousand dollars to the cost of each procedure. At almost the same time, the medical device community introduced a class of products called *stents,* tiny wire scaffoldings that hold coronary vessels open after the angioplasty is completed; these added several hundreds dollars to each procedure. More tellingly, the introduction of the drugs and stents broadened the overall indication for angioplasty, particularly among the sickest patients previously ineligible for *any* heart surgery. Per-patient costs are lower, especially over the short run, but aggregate costs to society because of the liberalization of the practice are higher. Although the new drugs and stents have both been shown to reduce the incidence of restenosis rates—necessitating that a percentage of those angioplasties be redone—the aggregate economic impact of these breakthrough technologies is additive, not cost-saving. The liberal use of both new technologies for most angioplasties to avoid the complications associated with a diminishing minority of the procedures represents better care at a higher combined cost. And the progress on angioplasty continues. In 2000 and 2001, researchers found strongly positive clinical findings associated with the additional use of intravascular radiation during an angioplasty procedure—yet another clinical gain for added cost that will marginally improve outcomes while aggravating the overall economics of a procedure performed on nearly a quarter of a million patients every year (*HCIA National Inpatient Profile,* 1992–1998).

Such technology-driven mixed news (good news clinically, bad news economically) comes out almost weekly in the war against cancer, and it invariably follows the same plotline. Breakthroughs in and broader mobilization of diagnostic technology allow doctors to detect various forms of cancer at progressively earlier stages, sending more people into treatment faster. A pair of illustrative clinical studies were published in 2000 regarding more aggressive use of colonoscopy to detect colon cancers. Both studies found that the standard diagnostic procedure, sigmoidoscopy, may "miss as many as one-third of all cancers or precancerous growths" (Becker, 2000, p. 52). The second study (Lieberman and others, 2000) concluded that "if patients were given a clean bill of health based on a sigmoidoscopy of the lower section of the colon, about half the cases of cancer or precancerous lesions in the upper reaches would be missed." Also according to the second study, which was published in the *New England Journal of Medicine* and widely reported in the popular media, "Colonoscopic screening can detect advanced colonic neoplasms in asymptomatic adults. Many of these neoplasms would not be detected with sigmoidoscopy" (Lieberman and others, 2000). Great news, right? It is unless you are an MCO, which pays on average $130 for a sigmoidoscopy versus $3,000 for a colonoscopy (Becker, 2000). Asymptomatic adults do not generate bills for MCOs to pay, beyond the cost of the now substandard sigmoidoscopy procedure. Those who *are* diagnosed with the disease, thanks to the now standard colonoscopy procedure, go immediately into expensive cancer treatment. A large group of people who a year earlier would have been health care consumers have thus metamorphosed into patients, an expensive change indeed. Once again, better medicine and bigger dollars, especially in the aggregate.

This metamorphosis now occurs faster than it ever did in the past, for one simple reason: the consumer health care information revolution. Before the onslaught of media coverage dedicated to medical news, and before widespread discovery of the Internet, demand among those asymptomatic adults for the more expensive, more invasive diagnostic procedure may have taken years to build to critical mass, because of the traditionally slow diffusion of new practice patterns among the physician community. Today, that demand will go into overdrive, as patients at risk for colon cancer tell each other about it electronically or discover it on health care Web sites. Colon cancer is highly hereditary, and patients with a family history of the disease know full well they need to be screened annually. In pre-Internet days, this was something Dr. Chang told them about and then did, using whatever diagnostic technique she was comfortable with and the health insurer would pay for. But as those same patients participate in Web-based discussions about their common medical concern—as they receive messages from "listservs," or see them posted on electronic bulletin boards, or e-mail them to each other—word about the better, more expensive procedure will spread like wildfire among motivated consumers. As a result, Dr. Chang will start sending these patients to gastroenterology specialists for colonoscopies—instead of performing sigmoidoscopies herself in her office—much more quickly than she would have had these studies come out ten years ago instead of today.

While we improve the quality of clinical care at the margins for heart disease and cancer, the third biggest killer in society—stroke and other brain-related disorders—is still mostly uncharted territory. As a result, dozens of drug and medical device companies have focused significant research and development on new clinical approaches to this major, and still only crudely addressed problem. Even more crudely addressed, though widely medicated, is depression, perhaps the most prevalent disorder in the United States if it were estimated accurately. Pharmacological and psychotherapeutic treatment of depression still focuses, respectively, on brain chemistry and cognitive patterns downstream of the real neuropathophysiology driving depression. Getting to the true roots of this widespread clinical problem is not cheap, and yet it proceeds. A good example of this progress was reported widely in the popular media in 2000. A group of researchers successfully adapted the microelectronics of cardiac pacemakers to treat depression at its source: the wiring of the human brain.

"Originally designed and used to treat epileptic seizures," reported the *Associated Press*, "the stimulator sends pulses to the brain stem through the vagus nerve, which stretches through the neck near the carotid artery. The pulses usually last about 30 seconds and occur every three minutes to five minutes. The stopwatch-size device is made from materials used in pacemakers and sits in the patient's chest with small wires leading to the vagus nerve" ("Doctors Test . . .," 2000). Here, an expensive technology developed for and used commonly in one sphere of medicine, at a predictable rate and cost, is applied to a completely different sphere, at a rate and cost unanticipated by anyone. As expensive as so-called talk therapy and drugs like

Prozac may be given the size of the afflicted population, their cost is a pittance compared with the potential aggregate cost of manufacturing and implanting these devices, should further clinical investigation warrant their elevation to a national standard of care.

The MCO culture of just saying no runs headlong into these kinds of medical breakthroughs every day. In the process, it also runs headlong into a broader cultural fact about American life: we will not accept no for an answer when our lives—our hearts *or* our minds—are at stake. Individual demand for immediate, unfettered access to ever higher quality, ever more expensive medical care is enshrined in our culture and defended aggressively by our legal system. Back in 1993, when biotech company Genentech was finally able to prove that its bioengineered clot-busting drug, Activase, improved mortality for heart attack patients by all of 1 percent (on an absolute basis), the drug, at $2,000 more per dose than streptokinase, its competing alternative, saw its market share increase from 50 to 66 percent. This shift in market share is particularly remarkable if you think back to 1993, when the nation's desire to control medical inflation had reached the point of obsession; employers en masse were buying into the MCOs' cost-effectiveness arguments; and managed care was not only the panacea for the Medicare and Medicaid programs but also served as the cornerstone for the Clinton plan for reforming the entire system. So why did Activase get a run-up in market share? Because the health care industry is *not* the medical industry, a problem explored in the next chapter. All the energy expended in administrative, policy, and business spheres on health care reform in 1993 was independent from and ignorant of actual medical practice, the same as it is now.

Back in 1993 while the nation's MCOs were gearing up to micromanage everything physicians like Dr. Chang did, she and her colleagues were quietly going about the business of diagnosing and treating patients, including increasing their relative use of Activase at a marginal cost of $200,000 per one hundred heart attack patients to save one additional life. Physicians willfully chose the leading-edge drug at ten times the cost of its cheaper alternative, despite the efforts of the MCOs, because to do otherwise would be to practice clinically substandard medicine for individual patients. As a culture, then and now, we would never tolerate such a thing, and our lawyers will make certain we never have to. From the cost-effectiveness or ROI perspective that defines the economic *ethos* of managed care, a puny 1 percent improvement in heart attack mortality for an ultimately disabling condition does not justify that additional $2,000 cost per patient.

Which begs the most unpleasant of questions: Which American heart attack patient will volunteer his or her life for the cause of cost containment? Our medical system is a mess for the same reason our roads are. We are a nation of fiercely independent, demanding individuals; we are permanently stuck in rush-hour traffic, one passenger per vehicle, and we wouldn't have it any other way. Popular debate over whether we should scrap the entire private insurance system and move to a single-payer model always boils down to one observation about how the system works in Canada: *they* ration care, and *they* have to wait in line for surgery. The MCOs also practice rationing, though they never call it that, and look how well that has worked. As the MCOs and the government struggle with ways to pay for a continuous flood of new medicines and clinical breakthroughs, the medical research community continues to churn them out and the media spreads the good news.

Sorting through today's medical breakthroughs is a big task competing for the attention of the MCOs' thousands of medical directors. This is especially difficult considering how they spend the bulk of their time, namely, coping with the day-to-day task of approving or denying payment for the basics and for *last* year's breakthroughs. According to a report in the *New England Journal of Medicine,* "A medical director at a large national HMO focused the company's quality-improvement efforts on five areas of clinical care: treatment of diabetes, treatment of congestive heart failure, care after myocardial infarction, treatment of depression, and women's and children's health. Because these quality-improvement initiatives cost money, they had to be approved by the organization's executive officer" (Bodenheimer and Casalino, 1999). This takes us back to the main argument made earlier in this chapter: in trying to improve care, the medical armies within the MCOs are subject to the accounting armies.

How do those in the MCO medical armies cope with this challenge? If the *New England Journal* analysis is accurate, they do so through systematic self-delusion. "In an effort to resolve these conflicts, medical directors have developed an ideology centered on the belief that high-quality care is less expensive than care of lower quality" (Bodenheimer, 1999). This naivete may be the result of their lack of training, which generally involves both medical and business school; neither program provides rigorous study of the epidemiology, public health, or medical economics disciplines that are at the heart of what they are trying to accomplish. In the work hours left over after second-guessing Dr. Chang's clinical decisions, medical directors seek to improve population health through programs that promote wellness, prevention, and disease management. The rest of their organizations are in the business of paying for these things, most of which are not "cost-effective" and never will be.

Consider the following example of how badly most of these numbers shake out. In 1999, Kaiser released a study showing that pneumococcal pneumonia in infants is preventable with a new vaccine. They tested the vaccine on nineteen thousand newborns, and it prevented the infection in all but one child. By contrast, in Kaiser's control group of the same size, thirty-nine children contracted the pneumonia (Lieu and others, 2000). The effectiveness of the new vaccine is great news—for everybody except Kaiser's accountants. Let's assume the four-shot regimen costs as little as $50 per infant. (Following much negative press about the vaccine's price, originally set at $150, the vaccine's maker backed down on the price, and as of this writing reliable pricing data is not available.) At $50 per vaccinated child (which excludes clinical administration costs) the total cost to an MCO for nineteen thousand infants is $950,000. The costs associated with the thirty-nine children contracting pneumococcal pneumonia, assuming a mean cost of $5,200 per illness, is $202,800. For the eyeshades running today's highly price-competitive MCOs, the new immunization program has a *negative* return on investment of 4.7. The nearly unique social orientation of Kaiser's not-for-profit mission will probably compel the organization to pay for these vaccinations, to its own financial detriment; the more common mission of all its competitor for-profit MCOs will probably compel them *not* to pay for these vaccinations.

There are exceptions to this rule, in particular flu shots and childhood vaccines for more common illnesses. But because such analyses stack up wrong for nearly every other aspect of preventive care, the nation's MCOs have no vested interest in managing anyone's health. Dr. Chang certainly has no interest in bearing the costs of preventive care, a source of enormous professional conflict for any good doctor. The only people with that vested interest are Dr. Chang's patients, or in the case of the Kaiser study, the parents of those thirty-nine children. The Twaddle Echo Factor would argue that employers of those parents also have an interest, considering what a child hospitalized with pneumonia means for workplace productivity; but as I pointed out in Chapter Two, there are numerous impediments to employers ever connecting these dots.

This is why we as a nation have two choices. We can decide to pay the added freight associated with higher quality health care and choose a Kaiser, which can pay that freight out of what the for-profit MCOs pay their shareholders. Or we can take back control from the MCOs altogether for our own medical coverage, purchasing either better insurance or paying Dr. Chang out of our own pockets for the preventive care she wants to deliver. Managed care exists because a large segment of the insurance market wants more affordable coverage and is only now beginning to realize what this affordability entails. *Somebody* has to subsidize the costs for all our medical progress. In health care, as in everything else in life, you get what you pay for.

CHAPTER 4

The Health Care Jobs Program

I n a large, windowless conference room in the basement of Community General Hospital, a twenty-five-year-old consultant stands at the end of the table, working through a PowerPoint presentation splashed across a rumpled screen. Along one side of the table sit the hospital's fifty-five-year-old CEO, two women from the marketing department, a managed care contracting manager, an analyst from the finance department, the administrator of the nephrology department, and an administrative intern. Across from them sit two contracting managers, a marketing manager, a program consultant, and an administrative intern from CareNet, the HMO that serves a portion of the state's Medicare beneficiaries. Two contract officers from the state's health insurance commission, one fidgeting, the other on the verge of sleep, sit in chairs along the wall. The room has the burnt-black smell of old, simmering coffee.

The hospital takes care of more than half of all patients included in CareNet's end stage renal disease program. The consultant is describing the details involved in the hospital's "carving out" of that program on a per patient per month basis.

"So we assume all the financial risk," the hospital's analyst asks. "Not just for the dialysis and the admits, but for all the drugs, labs, and nutritionals?"

"That's right," the consultant says.

The analyst turns to the nephrology department administrator. "Is that a big deal?"

"It's hard to tell," she shrugs. "I guess it depends on which ones fall in the bucket. Many of these patients are on a lot of meds—drugs for diabetes and heart disease—things like that." She looks down at the contract attachment on the table. "It's kind of hard to tell if this list covers all of them." She looks up from the paper. An uncomfortable silence fills the room. "Maybe we should have invited a doctor to the meeting."

Another uncomfortable silence.

The hospital's CEO leans forward in his chair. "Let me ask you all a basic question." He looks up at the consultant, over at his staff, then back to the consultant. "If we're at risk for all this stuff, but we have to pay the state back everything past a 4 percent margin, why are we even doing this?"

The consultant looks up at the presentation on the screen. "Because, uh, because that's the way it's going in ESRD contracting." He looks at the people from CareNet. "Right?"

"Absolutely," says one of CareNet's contracting managers, turning to CareNet's program consultant. "Right?"

"It sure is," he says. "That's the way it's going for hospitals with big ESRD volumes."

The CEO looks back at the consultant. "And you personally think this makes sense from a business perspective? I mean—we have to add the outpatient capacity, buy another dialysis machine, and figure out how to integrate all that outpatient drug information. That's a lot of money, a lot of stuff to do, a lot of risk."

"Yes, it is," the consultant says. "But the head of our health care practice and all the senior health care partners say it's the right thing to do. We have hospital clients in more than fifteen cities doing this. And they're making it work."

The CEO lets out a long sigh. "OK then." He perks up, turning to his staff. "Let's look at the contract."

Health care in America is a sizable and growing middle-class jobs program. Tens of thousands of well-meaning people work throughout the health care system, none of whom ever see a patient or deliver any actual medical care. They preside over an infinity of rules, regulations, forms, processes, contract outsourcing, financial brokering, benefit plan tinkering, analytical processes, incompatible data systems, and dead forests of paperwork. Health care administration in America is a Tower of Babel that reaches to the moon, built over decades specifically to cope with a "system" designed by historic accident, regulatory redundancy, and ever more ingenious entrepreneurial ambitions. The recurring impulse among everyone who tries to simplify and clarify the U.S. health care system is to dream up a business scheme that ultimately complicates and obfuscates it further. The result of every attempt at reform is the creation of more jobs.

Perhaps this is what we really want. Health care currently employs 17 percent of the U.S. workforce. Predominantly upper-middle-class jobs at Community General Hospital, CareNet, and the consulting firms that serve both are more prestigious and lucrative than predominantly middle-middle and lower-middle-class jobs cleaning up our cities, schools, and prisons. In many small and medium-size towns, a local hospital is the largest local business; this goes a long way in explaining why half the nation's hospital beds have been empty for decades. This outsized infrastructure is the result of government policies enacted back in the 1940s and 1960s designed specifically to create more hospital capacity. The government inadvertently continues to subsidize this health system redundancy by funding excess hospital-based specialties in its attempt to care for the uninsured. Because of the many health care market failures outlined earlier in this book, this overcapacity has simply been absorbed by the system, through misallocation and overutilization of resources, and through price inflation.

Among the many paradoxes of the health care industry, none has been more perplexing than the one affecting the law of inpatient supply and demand, as played out in the Community General Hospitals across the country. Under the faulty market economics of health care, the greater the supply of hospital beds, the higher the total hospital bill for the community. This inversion of normal market functioning is based on perverse collective clinical behavior observed for years across the industry: hospital bed supply drives demand, not the other way around (Starr, 1982). This problem applies not only to hospital beds but to the presence of excess big-ticket medical technology, large concentrations of specialists, and other costly resources like the dialysis machine that Community General will add after it and CareNet reshuffle the local ESRD patient population. That extra dialysis machine is the embodiment of what many refer to as the "medical arms race" in local health care markets across the country. One hospital purchases an MRI, as a competitive response so do all the other hospitals of its size in the market, and suddenly there is a concerted effort across the market to cover the enormous fixed costs of all the machines by using them. Without normal marketplace checks, hospital competition serves only to make the situation worse; more supply induces still more demand. As Nguyen and Derrick note in *Integrated Health Care Delivery,* "Increased hospital competition is associated with higher costs, lower occupancy rates, reduced efficiency, and more service offerings" (Nguyen and Derrick, 1996). So much for competitive market forces fixing the U.S. health care system.

The problem of hospital overcapacity was created by the government in the 1940s, when it attempted to alleviate an acute shortage of hospital beds with the usual federal medicine—more money. This was a shortsighted effort that created a chronic disorder far more destructive than the one it was meant to cure. In response to the perception that the United States had too *few* hospitals, the government bankrolled the Hill-Burton program in 1947, which was meant as a temporary boost to sagging capacity in selected areas of the country. Like most things involving government money, what was supposed to be extraordinary became expected; the medicine designed to relieve spotty symptoms became an addictive drug for empire-building state health officials and hospital administrators. The law aimed to set a ceiling on hospital beds at 4.5 per one thousand people, which was higher than most states at the time, and this ceiling eventually came to serve as the standard (Starr, 1982). As with defense spending, government funding in health care translates into one thing: more jobs.

Excessive expansion of hospital capacity development under the Hill-Burton program persisted until it was finally supplanted by an even greater aggravation to the problem, the introduction of Medicare in the mid-1960s. To win the support of the hospital lobby, the federal Medicare program included capital reimbursement for new hospital construction. This involved millions of dollars in government spending on new inpatient capacity and distorted what would almost certainly have been the marketplace's preference to develop lower-cost, outpatient capacity. Although government subsidies are usually at the root of numerous industries' overcapacity and resource misallocation—ranging from agricultural price supports to antiquated mining rights laws—health care seems particularly prone to this phenomenon. The result of decades of Hill-Burton—and faulty Medicare reimbursement schemes, which persist to this day—is a nation of five thousand hospitals, half of which sit idle, subsidized by artificially high prices charged for the patients in the other half (*Comparative Performances of U.S. Hospitals,* 1992–1998).

Natural market pressures to "rightsize" hospital capacity through aggressive pricing and utilization management by the MCOs are forever being thwarted by community efforts, hospital-building ambitions, and labor protests. This is particularly true in small towns with struggling local economies. A good example is the experience of one hospital in Fairfield, Alabama. As reported in *Modern Healthcare,* the town's mayor "wasn't about to let 80-year-old Lloyd Noland Hospital and Health System and its 600 jobs die. The hospital's owner had said that if it couldn't sell the 222-bed facility by September 30, it would close it. Hours before the deadline the city's Fairfield Health Industry Authority ponied up $10 million and promised another $11.2 million in renovations and working capital" (Taylor, 1999, p. 26). A different version of exactly the same story plays out every few months somewhere in the United States, usually a small town or inner-city neighborhood. The hospital slated for closure, its local advocates always argue, is a major source of jobs.

The same health care jobs program effect inspires the construction of new hospitals as frequently as it precludes the closure of old ones. Despite a persistent 50 percent occupancy rate for most hospitals, and the systematic shift of inpatient surgeries and other care to outpatient settings, new hospital construction proceeds apace, creating hundreds of design, construction, consulting, and support jobs in a community, all funded by public money either directly, indirectly, or eventually through higher health care costs. How much money are we talking about? The highly disputed new Cook County Hospital in Chicago will cost $626.3 million, after adding in the cost of new medical equipment and information technology. In a criticism of the controversial new construction, *Modern Healthcare's* editor, Clark Bell, noted that "the sad part is that those involved couldn't come up with a better strategy than a $626 million public works project" (Bell, 2000, p. 22).

The health care jobs program effect is strengthened daily because, just like the jobs program administered by the Pentagon, the government still purchases half of all medical care. This is why the industry's financial fortunes rise and fall with the budgetary whims of Congress. The most recent example of how this works was the roller-coaster ride that hospitals took after the passage and then modification of the Balanced Budget Act of 1997. After the act went into effect, "it took a little while for the federal reimbursement cuts to reach hospital company bottom lines, but when they did, they hit hard. Earnings suffered, which pushed stock prices down throughout the industry. At the end of 1999, Congress passed a roughly $16.1 billion federal reimbursement relief package, restoring some of what had been cut in 1997. . . . Hospital chains are reaping increases in federal Medicare reimbursements . . . helping them achieve and overshoot earnings targets" (Kirchheimer, 2000b, p. 81). This is consistent with Havighurst's broader observation that "Medicare's most significant side effect was to make the health care sector an arena for profit-seeking activity more than ever before. For the first time, hospitals and physicians could expect to be paid well for much of the care they had previously provided for less" (Havighurst, 2000, p. 89).

The complex matrix of health care purchasing—by the federal government through Medicare, by states through Medicaid, and by all the third, fourth, fifth, and counting, parties hired by employers—makes it impossible to fix this essential market failure. When Community General Hospital starts losing money on its harebrained new ESRD risk-contract, it will subsidize these losses by cranking up prices or utilization for patients elsewhere in its payer mix, such as those in the traditional Medicare program, commercially insured patients, and perhaps patients from CareNet itself. As a consequence, the whole capacity problem never gets fixed. More chaos, more inertia.

When government and private payers attempt to align their efforts at fixing the problem, Community General Hospital will resist mightily. A good example of this was the rare political alliance forged between MCOs and hospitals when the federal government attempted to introduce competitive pricing for Medicare beneficiaries covered under managed care risk contracts. The MCOs did not want the challenge to their profitability and administrative overhead that competitive pricing represented, and the hospitals did not want the payment squeeze downstream as the MCOs attempted to maintain that profitability and overhead. "It is hard to see how demonstrations such as this can ever be successful without having at least a dampening effect on the rates that plans pay to hospitals, physicians, and other providers," commented Barbara Cooper in her *Health Affairs* analysis of the competitive pricing demonstration project. "So it is not surprising that providers worked with the plans to kill the demonstrations" (Cooper and Vladeck, 2000, p. 53).

This political behavior is consistent with Clayton Christensen's observation, in the *Harvard Business Review,* that "powerful institutional forces fight simpler alternatives to expensive care because those alternatives threaten their livelihoods. And those opponents to low-cost change are usually lined up three or four deep" (Christensen, Bohmer, and Kenagy, 2000, p. 103). His comments go well beyond the walls of the hospital to refer to a broader phenomenon: "Our medical schools and residency programs have churned out specialists and subspecialists with extraordinary capabilities. But most of the things that afflict us are relatively straightforward disorders whose diagnoses and treatments tap but a small fraction of what our medical schools have prepared physicians to do. Similarly, the vast majority of research funding from the National Institutes of Health is aimed at learning to cure diseases that historically have been incurable. Much less is being spent on learning how to provide the health care that most of us need most of the time in a way that is simpler, more convenient, and less costly" (p. 104). Why? Because of the health care jobs program effect. Those high-tech, big institutional forces that have come to define the U.S. medical system create far more jobs per patient—that is, all those people in the meeting at Community General—than do primary care physicians working in modest community care settings.

THE MANAGED CARE JOBS PROGRAM

The number of CareNet people attending the Community General meeting illustrates another phenomenon: the health care jobs effect is equally pervasive in the MCOs, if not more so. The 80 cents of the premium dollar typically spent on actual medical care by commercial MCOs leaves 20 cents for executives to create jobs. How much money does this really entail? A window into the magnitude of this figure opened when a major national MCO unwound one of its biggest job-generating activities, the "utilization management" of routine patient care. "By scrapping its pre-approval process, United Healthcare freed up roughly $110 million in annual administrative expenses and trimmed its operating cost ratio to 16.8% from 17.1% a year ago" (Benko, 2000, p. 2). This was a deft public relations move, designed to counter growing public awareness of what MCOs actually do with our health care dollars. Most telling about the move was the fact that no other MCO followed United's courageous lead. This $110 million represents a sizable number of health care jobs; it also represents a sizable amount of turf for empire-builders within an MCO who, like most people in large organizations, define their career success not in terms of what they know or do but rather in terms of how many people they control.

The sheer number of dollars in play helps explain the bizarre, counterintuitive trend in administrative costs for MCOs since capturing much of the private health insurance market and engaging in an orgy of mergers and acquisitions. From 1987 to 1993, a period "in which managed care enrollment soared, private health insurance administrative expenditures per person covered rose by 236 percent, while HMO premiums rose 71 percent," writes Kip Sullivan in *Health Affairs* (2000, p. 143). These cost trends run counter to what every other industry experiences as it grows in market share and consolidates. "In most industries a doubling of production leads to a fall, not a large rise, in per unit administrative costs," he goes on to point out (p. 143). His same study found that "Minnesota HMOs increased their administrative spending per member by 403 percent . . . while their spending per member on medical care rose only 255 percent" (p. 143). This is more hard evidence of how money earmarked for medicine is siphoned off at an increasing rate by people who do not make that medicine, or prescribe it. MCO administrative costs do not go up relative to medical costs because it makes any sense; those costs go up because they make jobs.

It is easy and somewhat disingenuous to blame this collective rise in administrative costs solely on the greed and empire-building of those running the nation's MCOs. There are two other culprits, and the MCOs are helpless against both. The first major culprit, and the one that has allowed this problem to persist for so long, is the essential market failure of the private U.S. health insurance system. With so many commercial parties standing between what the MCOs offer in terms of price performance and those ultimately paying the price in lost cash wages, the MCOs are perfectly free to pursue their job-creation programs. The other big culprit is the utter complexity of the system, a vicious cycle of managed care business actions and public policy and legal reactions. More chaos, more inertia, more jobs.

Because MCOs do not deliver what they have promised, we respond with an ever growing tangle of regulatory burdens, at both the federal and state levels, to make them deliver at least some of it. This forces them to add more administrative tasks to their already overflowing to-do lists, and still more costs to their already considerable administrative overhead. The imposition of employers into the system, seeking always to balance their own financial pressures against demands from their employees, serves only to exacerbate the situation. Employers fiddle—one by one—with benefit plan designs to fill in gaps the regulators have missed or have not gotten to yet. This vicious cycle of health benefits give-and-take-and-give-back—imposed by fifty-one regulatory bodies and thousands of self-insured employers—represents an endless series of temporary solutions that only make the original problem worse. More demands, more administrative jobs, fewer dollars left over for actual medical care, and more demands in response to those diverted medical dollars. The cumulative effect of this vicious cycle is exponential, and it drives yet another health care jobs program. This particular one—perhaps one of the most lucrative on a per job basis—employs tens of thousands of lawyers, accountants, auditors, brokers, and consultants of every stripe charged with sorting out the whole mess. They too siphon off medical dollars into administrative buckets, and ultimately make the mess that much bigger and messier.

If we want to reverse course and spend more of our health care dollars on actual medical care, then we need to simplify the entire so-called health care system in the most basic and profound ways. Rather than shuffling the ESRD population back and forth between CareNet and Community General, we should address the fundamental reasons why both organizations have such bloated cost structures in the first place. If we do that, we will free up more than enough money to offer those patients real choices about where they get their medical care, not newfangled delivery systems they do not understand and that will not last anyway. This is why all attempts at reform should focus on fixing what created the Tower of Babel and its administrative jobs program in the first place: the sprawl of uncoordinated regulations at the federal level and across fifty states, tax-code incentives that stick employers and the government in the middle of everything, an endless proliferation of benefits plans by employers and government agents, and the financial rewarding of brokers and countless other middlemen for presiding over the whole disaster.

LIFE ON THE HOSPITAL CHAIN GANG

What about the other people in that meeting at Community General Hospital? Who are they and what are their professional lives like? Some of the biggest victims of the impossible problems wracking the U.S. health care system, aside from patients denied needed care and physicians frustrated daily in their attempts to provide it, are the hard-pressed people who run our hospitals. Community General's CEO and his staff are besieged on all sides by, among others

- Armies of contracting and other administrators from CareNet and a dozen competing insurers in its market
- Self-insured employers second-guessing all those insurers' premiums, pricing, and utilization data
- State and federal contracting officers, auditors, and agents
- Reporters looking for human interest scandals
- Financiers looking to buy or sell the hospital like a trading card
- Consultants selling the latest, billable business schemes
- Hundreds of frustrated physicians
- Anguished families, and their lawyers

How else can we explain the unparalleled level of job dissatisfaction among people engaged in what should be some of the most important work anyone could ever do? When surveyed in 2000, 40 percent of hospital administrators said they would "choose a profession other than healthcare if they could start their careers over, and 38 percent said they would not recommend healthcare to young students" (Jaklevic, 2000a, p. 40).

This is indeed a sorry state of affairs, and it does not bode well for the future of the hospital business. Job dissatisfaction this prevalent and profound guarantees that the kind of talent we need most in health care is increasingly likely to go elsewhere, leaving us with aging ranks of uninspired people to preside over hugely complicated organizations. It also explains the hospital industry's general lack of innovation and creativity in solving some of its most pressing problems. One commentator in *Modern Healthcare* went so far as to call what afflicts U.S. hospital management "courage anemia," attributing it to "management by inertia, which inhibits action and innovation" (Kazemek, 2000, p. 36).

As the U.S. health care nonsystem grinds on, what we get instead of courage, action, and innovation in hospitals is more of the same old thing.

The typical hospital today is run by either an academic lifer, a career administrator, an aging nun, or a middle manager who has spent his or her career working in the same small circle of hospital chains, based in faraway cities, with a changing kaleidoscope of corporate names. All are specialists in surviving the status quo, fighting daily battles with insurers, coddling physicians, and coping with reams of government and private reimbursement rules. Their every business move, designed to navigate the twin threats of financial insolvency and government prosecution, is mulled over for months with lawyers and consultants, and wrapped in layers of butt-covering paperwork.

I would venture to guess that those hospital job dissatisfaction statistics are so high not because the actual jobs are so awful. Rather, I believe (and have had numerous hospital CEOs admit to me) that their jobs cause intolerably high levels of professional *disappointment*, a collision of once-hopeful expectations with reality. Running Community General Hospital should be joyous, purposeful work. Its administrators preside over the staging area for the community's greatest dramas, a bustling facility where babies are born, traumas are quelled, medical breakthroughs are tested, new doctors are trained, and millions of people fight for their lives. The desire to participate in such dramas brought many hospital administrators into the profession in the first place. It is testament to the pressures and problems of the broader system in which our hospitals operate that so many have lost that inspiration.

Running a hospital is also economically critical work. The highest cost component of our health care system has always been and will always be inpatient care. Although three-quarters of all medical encounters occur in outpatient settings, inpatient encounters are the costly ones, consuming nearly 40 percent of annual health care costs in the United States every year. In their mobilization of the technological marvels that drive the modern health care system, U.S. hospitals are the embodiment of the greatest paradox of that system: they enable the most astounding feats of medical progress, while choking on the most astounding administrative stupidities involved in financing and delivering that progress.

Because of the proliferation of these administrative stupidities, the typical U.S. hospital has devolved into a paralyzed bureaucracy that, despite handling hundreds of millions of dollars annually, more closely resembles the government agencies that feed it and the academic institutions that train its leaders than the flexible, responsive organization demanded by a functional marketplace. As I've mentioned elsewhere, U.S. hospitals fall into four different groups, each with its own unique culture: academic institutions with conflicting missions, not-for-profit hospitals run by religious orders with a different set of conflicting missions, nonreligious not-for-profit hospitals like Community General that are governed by community leaders, and groups of for-profit hospitals that are owned, if not operated, by a small number of musical-chair hospital corporations based in three southern cities. The heterogeneity represented by these four different hospital types doomed, almost from the start, the movement throughout the 1990s to "integrate" the clinical and business operations of small, stand-alone facilities competing in what has always been a fragmented hospital community. Attempts to integrate teaching and nonteaching hospitals, Catholic and secular hospitals, and for-profit and not-for profit hospitals into "systems of care" has proven nearly impossible because of these conflicting values and cultures. As a result, such systems create more bureaucracy, not less, and many have resulted in highly public failures. If the meeting between Community General and CareNet seemed a little crowded, imagine the situation if Community General were trying to build the same ESRD program in conjunction with the teaching and Catholic hospitals across town.

How did a decade's worth of attempts to integrate hospitals turn out to be, in most cases, complete disappointments? The consensus among the health care industry's leading pundits, most of whom have never actually worked in a hospital, is that the problem stems from poor leadership. Classic Twaddle Echo Factor. In criticizing hospital leaders for failing to lead, the pundits are doing exactly what W. Edwards Deming warned us never to do when trying to diagnose an industry's woes: blame individuals for systemic failures (Deming, 1982). By contrast, I would argue that if our health insurance system functioned anything like a real market—and if the government dragged its reimbursement systems into the 1990s, let alone the new century—then we could greatly simplify the task of running a hospital and its leadership would flourish. Blaming hospital leaders for their lack of courage amid the chaos of the U.S. health care system is blaming the victim.

As commercial managed care fails to deliver on its most important promises and the government continues to "manage" the care it purchases from hospitals through fear, intimidation, and a fraud-and-abuse rebate program, we will get only more of the same. In the meantime, those who know how to play by the rules will continue to run the game. In 1999, turnover among hospital executives was 10.6 percent, its lowest in nineteen years, and roughly *half* the 20 percent turnover rate among senior executives in other industries (Jaklevic, 2000a). The lack of turnover—and the broader institutional paralysis both driving and perpetuated by it—helps explain why, in the words of one observer, hospital management "throughout the industry on average is anemic and arthritic . . . too weak to get the job done, too inflexible to do it differently" (Sherman, 2000, p. 28). Still more blaming of the victim.

Perhaps we should blame the victim's lack of training. There is little professionalism in the ranks of hospital administrators, despite the enormous diversity of technical demands placed on them. According to one report, "Health care administration programs are not growing at the pace of other professional graduate programs, such as business administration" (Jaklevic, 2000a, pp. 38–39). One editorial writer identifies a "huge development deficit in healthcare where many managers are virtually management-illiterate. The situation is equally bleak among staff" (Sherman, 2000, p. 28). His point is well taken when considering the hard facts: in 1999, the average hospital worker received six hours of continuing education, whereas the average Starbucks employee received thirty-six hours.

Maybe we should blame the victim's boss. Although they handle all those millions of dollars, most U.S. hospitals are still managed, ultimately, by community boards of trustees. Many members of these boards have substantial business experience, having built and run banks, factories, stores, and other businesses in the community; many other members simply have a lot of money to donate to the hospital. Whether these characteristics are sufficient to prepare people to oversee the running of a modern hospital is suspect. The situation is worsened by board members who do not believe they need any meaningful preparation, including the one who commented in *Modern Healthcare:* "The best trustees know nothing about healthcare other than that they and their friends need it and how the CEO intends to provide it" (Arnold, 2000, p. 72).

The virulent ignorance and abdication of responsibility expressed here—which typify what I have personally encountered among hospital board members across the country—are at enormous odds with the complex reality of running today's hospital. "Everyone in health care knows that governance boards reflect the local needs and histories of their respective organizations and communities," writes Steven Johnson (2000, p. 48) in *Modern Healthcare.* "The really good ones, however, know the difference between effective boardsmanship and successful operational leadership. They demand the development of sound business plans and are not handcuffed by industry fads" (p. 48). It is the *lack* of well-informed board members that explains why so many hospitals, when they do attempt to innovate, tend to do so in lockstep with those industry fads. Community Hospital's ESRD carve-out program is one example among hundreds that have come and gone over the past decade.

As the meeting at Community General illustrates, the aging of hospital executives, low turnover, and lack of business courage make a hospital especially prone to pursue business strategies proposed, ironically, by consultants with *no* experience running a hospital. We would be hard-pressed to imagine a scenario more absurd than the twenty-five-year-old consultant, fresh out of business school, telling the fifty-five-year-old hospital CEO why he needs to embark on a risky and expensive ESRD venture. And yet we do not have to imagine it; it happens every day in hospitals across the country. The CEOs and administrative staffs of hospitals like Community General are too often the recipients of pure Twaddle Echo Factor, peddled for tens of millions of dollars by the nation's consulting companies. This explains why so many industry fads prove to be exactly that, and why so many fail almost as quickly as they are dreamed up.

OLD SOUTH, NEW SOUTH

The managerial amateurism, ossification, and occasional desperation of the not-for-profit community hospitals explain the longevity of the for-profit chains. Because I am writing a book and not a magazine article, I hesitate to list the names of the current chains and the number of hospitals that each currently owns. Why? Because the list will change several times over before this book even goes to print. As anyone who has read *Modern Healthcare* for several years knows, the hospital chains come and go with numbing regularity: they incorporate, raise capital, buy hospitals with that capital, swallow each other, spin hospitals off to other chains, and just as quickly fall apart. The only thing that ever changes are the names of the chains, some quaint, others cryptic, others downright indecipherable: Charter, AMI, Basic American Medical, NME, Quorum, Health Management Associates, Universal, New American, OrNda, Paracelsus, Community, Healthtrust, HCA, Columbia, and back to HCA. Collectively, these well-financed corporations shuffle a total of approximately eight hundred actual hospitals back and forth, and as a result those working in the individual facilities often cannot even tell you who owns them that year. (When I asked one clinical director about the hospital's current owner, she actually had to look at the pay stub in her purse to make sure.)

There are two constants in this bizarre cycling and recycling of hospital corporations. Almost all the chains are headquartered in the South, which explains their cliquishness and conformity. And almost all of the chains are formed, run, and re-formed by the same people from the same families: Frist, McWhorter, Massey, Eskind, Ragsdale, and a handful of their loyal lieutenants. These families have made piles of money rolling hospitals into chains, taking them public, watching their business fortunes decline, taking them private, fixing them up, and taking them public again. They are politically connected at the national level. And notwithstanding the presence of the country music industry, hospital companies constitute the biggest economic force in Nashville. Once again, the exceptions prove the rule. The first of the two largest and most financially successful of the chains over time has been Tenet, which is run by an outsider, Jeffrey Barbakow, and operated not in Nashville but in southern California. The second was Columbia, which was founded by another outsider, Richard Scott, whose successful intrusion into their midst infuriated not only Nashville's hospital family dynasties but also the federal government for his acumen at playing the game of hospital reimbursement better than anyone in those dynasties. (For my painfully detailed and opinionated analysis of what really destroyed Scott's hospital corporate creation, see "Paradigm Lost: Deconstructing the Columbia/HCA Investigation," published in the March-April 1998 issue of *Health Affairs;* Kleinke, 1998b.)

How inbred do the hospital chains get? Consider the following three examples, cited here only because they were making health care news at the time of this writing.

A new hospital chain called HealthMont was founded in 2000 by Timothy Hill, a former executive of the bankrupt New American Healthcare Corporation. He started HealthMont by buying four New American hospitals. A former internal audit supervisor at Healthtrust, Hill approached Clayton McWhorter, Healthtrust's founder, with the idea for the new chain. McWhorter put him in touch with Richard Ragsdale, a founder of Community Health Systems, who now sits on HealthMont's board (Kirchheimer, 2000b).

A second new hospital chain, LifePoint, was spun out of Columbia, which doubled in size when it merged with HCA, and just as quickly shrank when Richard Scott was run out of town by HCA's founders, who have since renamed it HCA, The Healthcare Company. According to a report in *Modern Healthcare,* "Many of the hospitals that make up LifePoint's portfolio were involved in a previous Frist spin-off. As part of Healthtrust-The Hospital Co., they have been in and out of the Columbia fold several times" (Kirchheimer, 1999, p. 26).

A third new hospital chain, Iasis, shows just how closely interlinked the chains can be. McWhorter was an initial investor in Iasis, "injecting about

$2 million in the hospital company and helping pave the way for a $200 million investment from New York venture-capital firm Joseph Littlejohn & Levy that enabled it to buy 15 hospitals" (Kirchheimer, 2000a, p. 52). Iasis, which operates fifteen hospitals, hired Michael French to run its Arizona and Florida division, which includes six hospitals. According to a report in *Modern Healthcare,* French is the "former president and chief executive officer of Charter Behavioral Health Systems, the Alpharetta, Ga.-based psychiatric hospital chain that filed for bankruptcy in February" ("Former Charter CEO . . .," 2000, p. 20).

What is the point of all this flipping of local hospitals back and forth, aside from providing lucrative employment for the army of bankers, lawyers, and accountants required to paper the deals? The chains seek to assemble and cultivate four important if mostly intangible assets: professional management, purchasing power, marketing strength, and working capital in a fragmented hospital industry badly in need of all four. But the constant pursuit of the fourth asset subverts the successful acquisition of the first three. As the chains end up functioning more like investment banks than stable corporations—trading local hospitals back and forth like playing cards, running themselves occasionally into bankruptcy, and resurrecting themselves in new public form—can they possibly achieve any of these other important business objectives? The result of the corporate ownership shuffle is organizational paralysis at the local hospital level. When a hospital jumps in and out of a different chain every few years, how can it join forces with its temporary partners to enter into long-term purchasing or marketing arrangements? How can a local hospital executive not related to one of the Nashville families be confident enough of his professional longevity to pursue a truly innovative business strategy, especially when he sees colleagues at other hospitals hauled into court by the government and disowned by the chains?

The constant changing of the ownership guard galvanizes the conflict and disconnect between an out-of-town corporate headquarters and what are essentially local service businesses. Anyone who has lived through a management takeover knows exactly what this does to the morale of the organization and its ability to recruit and retain good managers. With nearly

20 percent of the nation's hospitals run by the same handful of people in distant cities, is it any wonder that those in the industry's managerial ranks continue to age, cower, and say that they wish they had picked a different career? This syndrome goes a long way in explaining why the Catholic hospitals, despite a more complex mission and set of values, are able to compete successfully with the better capitalized, more professionally managed for-profit hospitals. In my years of negotiating information systems contracts with hospitals across the United States, I have come to one overriding conclusion about their management: the Catholic hospitals get their executive talent from the top of the nun class, the for-profits get their talent from the bottom of the MBA class. Community General beware.

SPOONFULS OF SUGAR

Among the many uncomfortable moments in the Community General meeting, one of the more telling was the nephrology department administrator's recognition that a physician who actually treats ESRD patients might have been helpful in the discussion. Forget the struggle between the nun and the MBA class; unfortunately for hospitals (and all of us), the nation's hospitals do not draw enough of their executive talent from anywhere in the medical school class. The managerial talent gap afflicting U.S. hospitals is exacerbated by the single biggest challenge involved in their day-to-day management: managing physicians who drive most of their costs but are usually not their employees.

In his landmark study of the history of the U.S. health care system, *The Social Transformation of American Medicine,* Paul Starr points out that hospitals and physicians have always depended on each other, with the balance of power generally tilting toward the physicians. "The hospitals needed the doctors to keep their beds occupied," he writes. "The physicians' authority with patients and their strategic position in the system represented a resource that gave them power over institutions" (Starr, 1982, p. 218). Much has changed in health care since the decades when this imbalance first began, but the imbalance itself has not.

Notwithstanding the ambitions of the nations' MCOs, medical services vendors, and Internet entrepreneurs, the primary relationship at the heart of the U.S. health care system has always been, and will always be, that between the physician and the patient. This is a sacrosanct part of our culture, reinforced by everything from medical malpractice law to popular TV portrayals of physicians as tireless patient advocates in a system chock-full of patient adversaries. MCOs, "disease management" companies, larger hospitals, and countless others, perhaps taking their cues from the massive health care business combinations of the 1990s, mistakenly assumed that health care was "corporatizing" like the rest of the U.S. economy in a way that would finally neutralize or marginalize to some degree the physician-patient relationship. That may be how contracts read and budgets are set, but in the day-to-day reality of patient care, it is pure Twaddle Echo Factor. As David Mechanic writes in *Health Affairs*, we spent the past decade believing that "the basis of trust can be transferred from individual doctors to organizations," just as "we trust that airlines, banks, communications companies, and other service organizations will hire competent and responsible personnel, without insisting on individual personal relationships." By contrast, Mechanic argues, "Most patients view their care primarily through their relationships with their physicians and place an exceedingly high priority on their doctors as their agents" (Mechanic, 2000, p. 103).

As a result, managing a hospital today still means managing an independent class of professionals accountable to patients first, patients' attorneys second, their personal incomes third, and the hospital fourth. This pecking order is highly problematic for hospitals. Because of their independent accountability and authority, physicians will forever hold a certain veto power over nearly every aspect of a hospital's daily operations. As stated in Chapter One, physicians remain for the most part nonemployees who have de facto control over nearly all of a hospital's line employees, but traditionally, have little vested interest in the hospital's success.

The economics and organizational challenges involved in running Community General Hospital compel its CEO and his staff to cope with this situation. A physician should not only have been present at the ESRD meeting but would have been able to give the hospital's staff a sneak preview, based on complex clinical realities involved in ESRD, of why the program would be an operational and financial disaster. Or maybe not. The point is that nobody in the room really knew. The success or failure of Community General's new ESRD program will depend for the most part on one thing: the ability of the hospital's physicians to make it succeed or fail.

There is tremendous financial leverage associated with the proper alignment of physician and hospital incentives. As one of many examples, hospitals for years have been struggling to standardize the purchasing and use of medical devices and supplies; the more successful they are at reducing product brand variety in a class of supplies—for example, the type of balloon catheters for angioplasty—the lower the hospital's per unit purchasing and total inventory costs for those supplies. Successful management of admitting physicians translates into better purchasing decisions, lower costs, and higher patient satisfaction. Physicians who are fully engaged in making these decisions, rather than having decisions imposed upon them long after meetings between consultants and hospital administrators have ended, are more likely to embrace those decisions. To follow the purchasing example, when interventional cardiologists practicing at a hospital participate actively in the selection of a standardized balloon catheter, they are much more likely to comply with this standardization. Such compliance translates into more predictable utilization, which in turn translates into significantly reduced supply costs.

Aligning physician clinical practices with a hospital's business strategies translates into even broader cost savings because it involves the standardization of medical *process* delivery, not just medical product selection. This is proven most obviously in its absence. As one observer notes, "Strategies and tactics that could produce significant gains for the organization often are not pursued for fear that physicians will 'go to war' over the change, such as clinical service consolidation and renegotiated contracts" (Kazemek, 2000, p. 36). Cognizant of the problems associated with this resistance, we have come to recognize that better hospital management involves primary leadership by the hospital's physicians, not by its professional administrators.

This homily, a rare instance when the Twaddle Echo Factor has actually gotten it right, is easier said than done. Physicians are forever mindful of who they are and where they came from, which makes them suspicious of even the simplest business reforms. Unfortunately for physicians, as they express skepticism or outright hostility toward a hospital's latest attempt to improve its clinical operations, they are undermining the power base they are trying so desperately to defend. As Mechanic notes in his *Health Affairs* analysis of how this power struggle is evolving, "Corporate medicine has taken from physicians much control over forms of organizational practice and payment, the uses of technology, and the division of labor. It does so with the assent of employers and government because it has demonstrated capacity to contain the growth of medical costs. Thus, the context of medicine has altered radically from what it was just a couple of decades ago" (Mechanic, 2000, p. 103).

But the context remains essentially the same, at least for those trying to make a hospital function more efficiently. The conventional wisdom that hospital leaders and their admitting physicians need to get along better rarely takes a full accounting of one of the most fundamental problems built into any modern health care system: *health care and medicine are not the same thing; each exists in a vastly different intellectual sphere from the other.* Health care and medicine are different technical disciplines, and the complexities of each erroneously presume the relative simplicity of the other. This helps explain why ready-made business solutions for hospital clinical departments—designed to improve profitability by cutting costs and peddled by the nation's so-called reengineering consultants—generally do not work. These solutions, like Community General's new ESRD program, hugely underestimate what it actually means to deliver care to complexly ill patients in those departments. Those delivering that care are just as frustrated; they in turn hugely underestimate the legal, financial, and organizational hurdles to throwing more money at a hospital department to improve quality. This situation is made worse by how those solutions are packaged and sold. The myriad consulting firms and information technology vendors who sell them tend to side with the administrators who pay them, not with the physicians who are the only ones who can successfully implement them in daily practice.

104

The chronic underestimating of the complexity of medicine by hospital administrators and their consultants provides fodder for physicians who are only too ready to chafe against every effort at fixing the hospital, no matter how earnestly intended. Meanwhile, the threat of medical malpractice lawsuits—with their permanent, toxic effects on a physician's career—does not help. I have never witnessed or heard of a consulting firm or information technology vendor willing to take on the resulting liability, if their reengineering strategies or clinical decision support systems produce a bad patient outcome. Always and forever, the legal liability flows back to the physician. This is one more reason why hospital business strategies that attempt to drive hospital clinical reforms often fail. Hospital administrators, consultants, information technology vendors, and most blatantly the managed care industry, are eager to reengineer medical care through new strategies, clinical-process tinkering, data systems, or reimbursement controls. But they abdicate any responsibility for what happens when these various health care business strategies result in bad medicine.

Considering all this, is it any wonder that 40 percent of the nation's professional hospital administrators express regret over their choice of career? Through this remarkable level of job dissatisfaction, they are, in part, expressing the enormous frustration that comes with trying to manage what they do not really understand. Is there a quick fix for this problem? No. There is an extremely slow fix, one that involves the development and sponsorship of intensive, interdisciplinary training in both medicine and health care that the current, aging generation of hospital administrators never had. The same thing needs to happen on the other side of the great divide: we need to train the next generation of physicians to be functionally literate in health care, not just medicine. Without the availability of this type of interdisciplinary training, those running Community General Hospital will never know enough about the complexities and nuances of medicine, and the physicians treating Community General's patients will never know enough about the complexities and nuances of health care.

As we attempt to reform the health care system in ways that make running a hospital less like playing a game of bureaucratic chicken with managed care and government payers and more like running an actual business, we need to fix the most basic management problem plaguing U.S. hospitals. The first and last steps in this process are to teach a new generation of administrators and physicians what the other actually does all day. This is nothing short of a mutual cultural revolution, one that will cultivate in both professions greater understanding of and respect for each other's incredibly demanding disciplines.

CHAPTER 5

Chaos in the Clinic

He who has health has hope,
and he who has hope has everything.

Arab proverb

Joe Olson, sixty-one years old with a ten-year history of heart disease and hypertension, has just committed suicide. To see how this happened, we need to go progressively backward in time.

Over the past year, Joe had been deeply clinically depressed. The first signs of his depression appeared a year after his heart surgery in 1997, a three-vessel coronary bypass graft procedure. Joe's extended convalescence from the surgery and the complications that followed led to an early retirement that he had never planned on taking. A few months before Joe retired, his wife was diagnosed with breast cancer and endured a six-month regimen of chemotherapy and radiation treatment. Joe blamed himself. A lifelong smoker, he had recently started smoking again in the presence of his wife, but never told his doctors. He also never admitted to them that he was not regularly taking the antidepressant one of them had prescribed.

Joe's depression and suicide might be attributed to what may have seemed overwhelming psychic and emotional stressors. Or could it be attributed to something else?

The heart surgery had been long and difficult, and was complicated by an ischemic stroke that occurred while Joe was recovering in the cardiac care unit the next day. Most multiple-vessel bypass procedures require clamping off the patient's aorta for up to several hours. The longer the surgery, the longer the aorta remains in the grip of the clamp. When the surgeon unclamps the aorta, microscopic blood clots known as *emboli*—built up during the procedure—are released from the aorta into the patient's arteries. They swirl like a galaxy of black stars through the bloodstream. Many emboli dissolve on their own, others eventually lodge in tiny vessels throughout the patient's body, and an errant few snag in the blood vessels of the patient's brain. Many researchers believe these emboli in the brain explain the cognitive decline and mood disorders seen in a large percentage of patients after bypass surgery. They may also explain a percentage of the strokes suffered by a small number of patients after the procedure.

If we were to dissect and examine Joe's aorta as part of an autopsy, we would find a barely perceptible structural anomaly: one side of the interior wall of his aorta is momentarily convex, whereas the walls of a normal aorta are fully concave. This subtle structural feature may have increased the number of emboli formed during Joe's bypass. Or he simply may have been unlucky when the normal number of emboli were released.

The slight abnormality in Joe's aortic wall formed seven and a half months before he was born. If this event that had occurred when Joe was still an embryo did in fact increase the number of emboli in his aorta during the bypass, then his depression and suicide in 2001 was an inevitable outcome of vascular cells multiplying in a less-than-perfect way in 1939. Or maybe not.

Chapter Four ended with a prescription for educating health care administrators about medicine and doctors about health care. A lesson central to both types of education is a hard, unpleasant, potentially disturbing one, and thus rarely taught to anyone. The odyssey of historic, policy, legal, technological, and cultural accidents that coalesced into what we have come to call our health care system all point to a single, profound, underlying fact of both health care *and* medicine: chaos is the exception, not the rule. Health care is a complex, fragmented, multidimensional system, wrapped around the discipline of medicine, which is itself enormously complex, fragmented, and multidimensional. As we toggle between the two, the effects of chaos grow on a seemingly logarithmic scale.

Unintended consequences plague nearly every aspect of running a hospital or practicing medicine. Many of them cannot be anticipated, controlled, budgeted for, or micromanaged away. Clinical experiences like Joe Olson's suicide typify the endless, nuanced ways that complexity plays itself out everyday in medicine and continues to confound physicians. Business systems that attempt to classify and judge the performance of Joe's providers are subject to their own version of the same bewildering technical problems confronted by those carrying out Joe's clinical postmortem. In this chapter, we will explore chaos theory—or what has come to be known as *complexity theory*—in the context of both medicine and health care. First, an important caveat. A disciplined, literal application of complexity theory to medicine and health care is well beyond the scope of this book, my scientific skills, and no doubt your patience. Credible versions of these applications would require two distinctly different books, both of which are begging to be written. In their absence, what follows in this chapter is a brief exploration of the tenets and applications of complexity theory as highly useful metaphors for the broader problems described in this book.

A few months after my book *Bleeding Edge* was published in 1998, I received an unsolicited e-mail from Dr. John Cook, a former industrial engineer turned physician. He had spent years running a busy hospital ICU, and at the time was engaged in trying to improve the clinical operations of a hospital in suburban Washington, D.C. Although generally supportive of many of the arguments I presented in the book, he was forcefully critical of my chapter on industrialization—my lengthy technical sermon on the promises of information technology and data analysis to reduce variations and unpredictability in medical care. In his e-mail, Dr. Cook introduced me to complexity theory. He wrote that this arcane and intriguing science was especially relevant to the realities of the clinic, and explained why medicine resisted the types of activities and efforts I was celebrating in my book (John Cook III, e-mail to the author, Sept. 1998).

I have since explored complexity theory at some length, with great intellectual delight. In the process, I have come to recognize that this relatively new scientific discipline not only has broad applicability to medicine but also explains why none of the easy answers in health care—managed care, the computerization of clinical processes, physician reimbursement reform, or other newfangled solutions—ever seem to work. Complexity theory argues that a fixed set of inputs will never produce a predictable set of outcomes, even when those inputs are seemingly held constant. Why? Because in the real world, there will always exist an infinite number of inputs that cannot be accounted for fully or held constant. The scientific method has, as it turns out, been "fudging it" all along.

For both the medical and health care systems, the emergence of an infinite number of potential outcomes looms ever larger and more perplexing as the science of medicine evolves and improves. Ironically, each medical success creates a plethora of more problems for both medicine and health care to solve. The astounding miracles of medical technology that we have brought into everyday clinical practice creates an ever widening set of practice variations, an older and more demanding population of people to take care of, and an ever greater likelihood of "bad" outcomes when we push increasingly fragile people through a bigger, more complicated medical machine. Surgeon and acclaimed author Sherman Nuland articulated this paradox in a *Wall Street Journal* editorial: "Patients and physicians are victims of the extraordinary success achieved by biomedical science in the past 40 years. Diagnostic and therapeutic methods that were relatively simple until the mid-1950s have become increasingly effective, but in the process they have also become increasingly complex, and sometimes formidably risky" (Nuland, 1999).

Consider the recent well-publicized medical errors report published by the Institute of Medicine, which claimed to have identified ninety-eight thousand preventable annual deaths in U.S. hospitals (Kohn, Corrigan, and Donaldson, 2000). The study was widely reported in the popular media, numerous politicians got good airtime decrying its findings, the managed care industry gleefully delivered a collective "I told you so," a hog's trough of public and foundation funding filled up quickly to study and "fix" the problem, and the usual harebrained business schemes followed just as quickly to feed at that trough. The ninety-eight thousand annual deaths reported make great headlines, as if they were ninety-eight thousand murder victims or—as countless people have pointed out from podiums and in print—passengers on the proverbial jumbo jet that crashes every day. Moral indignation mixed with money is a delectable brew for those who have always capitalized on health care's latest bad news, and the IOM was a bacchanal, an orgy of industry twaddle.

Time for a reality check. Yes, many of those deaths are attributable to illegible handwriting, incomplete paper charts, and medieval hospital information systems. But the real story behind the IOM report is far more complicated than the Twaddle Echo Factor would have it, and is nothing any patient wants to hear. Most of those ninety-eight thousand deaths are nobody's fault; they are the fault of an unwieldy system. No amount of media outrage, political grandstanding, or public pronouncements—nor any of the numbingly familiar, self-serving managed care or information technology solutions—will ever fix this problem. The IOM's findings may have shocked the nation, but they came as little surprise to people who actually understand medicine. As Dr. Nuland noted in his analysis of the study, "With so many steps and so many people involved in every aspect of care, the possibilities for error multiply, and small lapses quickly escalate into major events and occasionally into tragedies. Able and well-meaning personnel are caught up in a system filled with the possibility of misadventure, where the smallest error can have catastrophic consequences" (Nuland, 1999).

The "smallest error having catastrophic consequences" is the core tenet of complexity theory. This theory was developed back in 1961—most tellingly, by complete accident—through an experiment with a simple weather model (Gleick, 1987). With only a handful of weather variables in play in his model, MIT physicist Edward Lorenz saw the world of traditional science unravel. What should have been a mathematical replication of his earlier results, using virtually the same values for the same variables (he rounded numbers that went to the millionth decimal place down to the thousandth place), Lorenz's model produced a completely different outcome a few short clips into his modeled future. He began manipulating the least powerful of those variables and found that the slightest tweak produced very different results, almost immediately. It was the equivalent of God's spreadsheet crashing. Lorenz further found that the unpredictability of the model's outcomes, based on the slightest manipulation of input variables, unfolded in a predictable pattern. He called the artful, spontaneous patterns of unpredictability that emerged from his computer *nonperiodic flow*, a phrase later refined to *nonlinear dynamics*. His simple discovery of the exaggerated effects of rounding already small numbers represented a splintering—at a level approaching numeric infinitesimality—of both Newtonian physics and Cartesian mathematics, upon which our entire scientific tradition has been based. A terrifying new science was born.

Contemporary complexity theory has since grown into a diaspora of scientific pursuits. Each application flows from three interlocking principles: (1) a tiny disruption in a remote corner of some systems will be magnified throughout those systems and wreak havoc on their entire functioning; (2) the closer and closer we look for tiny disruptions, the more and more of them we find, until our perceptions have telescoped to an infinitesimal scale, and (3) the havoc that emerges does so through an ever more elegant patterning. The principles of complexity theory describe precisely what occurs throughout both medicine and health care, affecting nothing less than

- Many important and basic facts of biological processes
- Epidemiologic patterns of infectious disease and treatment resistance
- The clinical behavior of physicians
- Reactions of patients to their medical conditions and to their physicians' behavior
- Physician reactions to their patients' reactions
- The discovery of new medicines
- The clinical success or failure of those new medicines
- Reimbursement patterns for hospitals and physicians
- The health care purchasing behavior of employers and government

- The financing and functioning of managed care organizations
- The financing of Medicare

Given the pervasiveness and power of its effects in medicine and health care, complexity theory often serves to explain why so few solutions for both, whether regulatory or market-based, ever fix anything and in many cases actually aggravate the situation. There is simply no way to predict what will happen next in even the most seemingly isolated segment of a $1.3 trillion-dollar-per-year "system." Doing so is as intellectually daunting as trying to figure out why Joe Olson committed suicide. This is especially true when that system's daily landscape is peopled with millions of individuals, many in profound crisis; when it is continually disrupted by the introduction of new medical technologies; and when twenty thousand third parties try to micromanage the whole mess. James Gleick, the author who codified complexity theory in his brilliant, comprehensive, and highly readable 1987 book *Chaos,* was not specifically referring to medicine or health care when he wrote that "even when a damped, driven system is at equilibrium, it is not at equilibrium, and the world is full of such systems" (Gleick, 1987, p. 43). But he might as well have been.

HAVING A BAD O'HARE DAY

Gleick could also have been thinking of the nation's air transportation system, which provides us with an excellent analogy for how complexity theory works in the health care and medical communities. With its complex hybrid of private market forces and government regulation, its mix of expensive technology and large numbers of people, its highly skilled and often recalcitrant workers in the cockpit and its hard-pressed and often passive-aggressive workers in the trenches—not to mention its general unpleasantness for most consumers—the airline industry has always served as a useful metaphor for why the U.S. health care system is so screwed up. I have spent many a long evening at Chicago's O'Hare airport, with dozens of flights delayed because of a thunderstorm in Wichita or crew shortage in Dallas; thanks to complexity theory, I now know why. The breakdown of a major, busy airport because of an isolated weather event or equipment failure in a distant city is the embodiment of Gleick's observation that "a chain of events can have a point of crisis that could magnify small changes. Chaos meant that such points were everywhere. They were pervasive" (Gleick, 1987, p. 23).

Just as in health care, attempts by the government to fix marketplace failures in other industries through piecemeal legislation or mandates too often run the risk of accomplishing the exact opposite. Many have argued that airline deregulation in the 1980s is the root cause for a system on the perpetual verge of breaking down today. If so, then this cause and effect mirrors the way de facto deregulation of the U.S. health care market—through the use of commercial MCOs instead of a single payer to ration and contain costs—has grossly complicated, rather than simplified, the market's functioning. Consider the situation at LaGuardia, one of the nation's busiest airports and the one with the most flight delays. According to the *Wall Street Journal*, "LaGuardia has become the unlucky exemplar of air-traffic grid-lock precisely because of efforts by Congress and the Clinton administration to improve air service" (Brannigan, 2000). In 2000, Congress passed a law that "aimed to increase competition and expand service to smaller cities by lifting decades-old restrictions on flights in and out of LaGuardia and some other major airports," the *Journal* reported. "But the law yielded more than anyone bargained for as airlines added nearly 300 new flights at the smallest of New York City's three major airports with an already crowded roster of about 1,000 flights a day" (Brannigan, 2000).

As in health care and medicine, the complexity that rules our air transportation system feeds on the individual actions of millions of people, many of whom would rather be anywhere but stuck inside that system. The weather in Wichita may be fine, and yet I am sitting in O'Hare once again, this time because of a missed connection. Tonight, despite the government's efforts, my flight out of LaGuardia would have been on time. Unfortunately, a drunken passenger went into a rage at the flight attendants because he did not like his seat assignment and had to be forcibly removed from the plane by airport security; this held up our departure just long enough for an afternoon thunderstorm to roll in, stranding us on the runway for an extra half

114

hour. And so I miss my connection and spend another night eating Chinese fast food and browsing the newsstands of O'Hare, wondering if I will make it to Seattle at all for the next day's meeting—all because of one drunk. Isn't complexity theory fun?

I could have chosen a different set of flights from New York to Seattle. But that would have required my anticipating the actions of a drunken passenger, which, obviously, neither I nor the airline can do. Such anticipation would be akin to observing and quantifying an infinity of possible factors that affect an infinity of potential outcomes, a pure application of complexity theory. This is something that those trying to reengineer a hospital, medical practice, or population's health status cannot do any more readily than I can when I book my flights. In complexity theory, there is an infinity of variation that emerges to our senses as we move ever closer to the thing we are measuring. We experienced this phenomenon as we went progressively deeper into Joe Olson's medical history and physiology: we looked beyond the obvious psychological factors associated with his depression, and found the potential culprit in a few fetal vascular cells gone slightly awry.

FROM HERE TO INFINITY

In the language of complexity, the variations that emerge as we look more closely at the things we used to round off are pictorialized as *fractals*. Popular as colorful computer screen savers in engineering and computer science departments, fractals represent the endless splintering of reality across space and over time as we zero in on its surfaces. Fractals are described by Gleick as "faults and fractures" that so "dominate the structure of the earth's surface that they become the key to any good description, more important on balance than the material they run through" (Gleick, 1987, p. 105). Fractals describe the vagaries associated with treating unique and uniquely complicated patients like Joe Olson who, in toto, make up the "surface" of the health care system. They also often describe the most fundamental facts of biology. As Dr. Ary Goldberger writes in *The Lancet*, "non-linear systems with fractal dynamics (such as the neuroautonomic mechanisms regulating heart-rate variability) behave as if they were driven far from equilibrium under [even normal] conditions. This kind of complex variability, rather than a single homeostatic steady state, seems to define the free-running function of many biological systems" (Goldberger, 1996, p. 1314).

The human circulatory system is an elegant illustration of this phenomenon. Joe Olson's deep depression and suicide may not have been caused by the structural anomaly of his aorta and the formation of excessive emboli during the bypass. His death may ultimately have been caused by a normal number of emboli, streaming through his brain's blood vessels in a minute, random pattern that as yet cannot be predicted or controlled.

Such patterns occur throughout human anatomy. "Examples of fractal-like anatomies include the arterial and venous trees, the branching of certain cardiac muscle bundles, as well as the ramifying tracheobronchial tree and His-Purkinje network," Dr. Goldberger points out. "Mechanistically, these self-similar structures all serve a common physiological function: rapid and efficient transport over a complex, spatially distributed system. Fractal processes generate irregular fluctuations on multiple time scales, analogous to fractal objects that have a wrinkly structure on different length scales." The example Goldberger gives shows a "series of heart rates from a healthy individual plotted on three different scales. All three graphs have an irregular wrinkly appearance, reminiscent of a coastline or mountain range" (Goldberger, 1996). Thus, we return to Gleick's metaphor of the earth's surface, and how quickly it mutates before our eyes as we move in for an ever closer look. In a different article, Dr. Goldberger goes on to note that medical science has not coped with this well. "Sometimes the textbook approach seems to dance around the truth," he writes in *Biophysics Journal,* allowing the ambiguity included in a cornerstone medical text to speak for itself: "'In the gradual transition from one type of artery to another it is sometimes difficult to classify the intermediate region. Some arteries of intermediate caliber have walls that suggest larger arteries, while some large arteries have walls like those of medium-sized arteries. The transitional regions . . . are often designated arteries of mixed type'" (Goldberger, Bhargava, West, and Mandell, 1985, p. 525).

116

The presence of fractals and other descriptive tools of complexity theory abound in anatomy and physiology. They describe not only heart-rate variability but also "fluctuations in respiration, systemic blood pressure, human gait, and white blood cell counts" (Goldberger, 1996). But as the third principle of complexity theory is an empirical patterning of what defies simple, traditional linear equations, Goldberger finds hope in the fractals of human physiology. "If scale-invariance is a central organising principle of physiological structure and function," he writes, "we can make a general, but potentially useful, prediction about what might happen when these systems are severely perturbed" (Goldberger, 1996).

Predicting, budgeting for, and treating these "perturbations"—the real source of any disease, its sequellae, and its prognosis—is no small task. The intellectual challenges and rewards of doing this the right way tower over all the crude disease management tools and shrink-wrapped software designed and peddled with such enthusiasm to hospitals, physician groups, and MCOs. Credible versions of such tools, built on the principles of complexity theory, are a long way off, as far off as a true cure for cancer. Genomics research is the latest promise, heavily financed and promoted by Wall Street and its portfolio of bioinformatics companies. Thanks to the vividness and near-universality of the Twaddle Echo Factor regarding genomics throughout the industry, most actually believe that the recent unraveling of the human genome will allow us to target and cure various diseases at the level of the individual. But the scientific facts do not stand up to the business hype. We have known for several years about BRCA1 and BRCA2, two variations of the same gene that have been positively associated with breast cancer, and yet they accurately predict the disease only 45 percent of the time. Even the most sophisticated genomic data are imprecise thanks to, once again, the mischievous work of complexity theory at the level of cell biology.

The complexity at work in our most fundamental biological processes explains why we still cannot answer that most critical and perplexing of questions: Why is it that some people get cancer and others do not? As Dr. Gouri Passi asks in his essay on complexity theory and medicine in the

National Medical Journal of India, "Of the hundreds of people from a similar genetic pool and similar environmental exposures, why does one per chance develop cancer? Or going to a more microscopic level, of all the cells exposed to a similar internal milieu and with similar genetic material, why does one turn malignant?" (Passi, 1999, p. 93). The honest answer is: we do not have a clue. Why one person with a BRCA1 imperfection develops cancer and another does not remains as much a mystery as the real cause of Joe Olson's depression and death.

WHY IT IS CALLED MEDICAL "PRACTICE"

Physicians grapple with the effects of complexity theory in their daily practice. They recognize, if only subconsciously, that the principles of complexity that rule a patient's cells aggregate in even more unpredictable ways to rule that patient's diagnosis and prognosis. And so they suspend the laws of complexity, develop an intuitive sense of patterning, diagnose and treat patients consistent with that patterning, and leave the rest to chance. As Dr. Goldberger points out, "The practice of bedside diagnosis would be impossible without the loss of complexity and the emergence of pathological periodicities. It is these periodicities and highly structured patterns—the breakdown of multiscale fractal complexity under perturbed conditions—that largely allow clinicians to identify and classify many pathological features of their patients" (Goldberger, 1996, p. 1313).

In this sense, physicians attempt to strike a three-part intellectual compromise of sorts, combining an innate understanding of the complexity of a patient's physiology, an acceptance of certain constants based on their own pattern recognition, and a continual refinement of those patterns based on their accumulation of patient-by-patient clinical experience. The exquisiteness of this cognitive compromise defies codification, replication, or even explanation, really. And it belies why the best physicians always insist—despite the criticism and ambitions of others throughout the health care industry—that practicing medicine is indeed an art, not a science.

The cognitive challenges of combining complexity theory with clinical experience are infinitely more nuanced and complicated than any set of care

118

guidelines or utilization review process could ever incorporate. Despite the growing imposition of concurrent and retrospective clinical practice control systems by third, fourth, fifth, sixth, and seventh parties, physicians still rely on their own empirical knowledge and experience in their daily work. They are trained to observe the most subtle patterns—or the failure of those patterns—when diagnosing and treating patients. As Dr. Passi notes, "Experience has taught us which arrhythmias were likely to degenerate in ventricular fibrillation or cardiac chaos. But the underlying secrets about why some did and some did not, have yet to be unraveled" (Passi, 1999, p. 94). This explains why so much of medicine—notably critical care and cancer treatment, two of its most expensive components—involves intuition and trial and error. It also explains how and why even the most common medical practices can generate a host of good and bad unintended clinical consequences.

Though few oncologists would refer to what they do as practicing complexity-based nonlinear systems thinking, that is exactly how they approach the formulation of individual treatment regimens for individual patients. Nonlinear systems are, according to Dr. John Marshall, the "basis for the treatment of cancer, in which adjuvant therapy is designed to target the interactions of several interdependent biological processes, rather than a single one" (Marshall, 2000, p. 2648). Another good example is multiple organ dysfunction syndrome, a broad clinical description that describes much of what occurs in our nation's ICUs, consuming untold billions of health care dollars every year. In an editorial in *Critical Care Medicine* devoted to complexity theory's effects on this syndrome, Dr. Marshall concludes that "a stable state of 'chronic critical illness' is best understood through a consideration of the principles that govern complex nonlinear systems." He notes that a series of articles published in the same journal "provide a compelling argument that the critical elements of acute inflammation are not the individual proinflammatory and anti-inflammatory mediators, but the consequences of their interactions in concert. They have transformed the monotone of systemic inflammatory response and compensatory anti-inflammatory response into a glorious symphony of chaos" (Marshall, 2000, p. 2648). This "glorious symphony of chaos" resounds in our ears as we review Joe Olson's medical history and pathophysiology.

It also should provide, once and for all, the only explanation necessary for a stubborn feature of the health care system that has forever eluded legions of twaddle-echoing critics. Doctors practice medicine one patient at a time. This is how they are trained, and this is how they respond to data that purport to measure their outcomes.

"My patients are sicker," they holler back at the reengineering consultants, data analysts, and MCO number crunchers. "My patients are complicated, they do not speak English well, more of them are depressed, and a large number of them had problems with insurance coverage last year—and your data do not account for any of that!"

As much as health care administrators chafe at these objections—and as often as I have heard them derided by people throughout the managed care and health care information communities—they remain unassailable. Why? For one simple reason: the things in medicine we measure least often may be the things affecting cost and outcomes the most. In the case of Joe Olson, it may have been an embryonic event no one knew about or could have done anything about; all the physician browbeating and medication compliance rituals in the world may not have been able to save Joe's mind from an invasion of excessive aortic emboli.

The "rounding" problems that unleash complexity factors in the clinic, and that are never accounted for in provider performance measurement systems, do not apply to every type of medical study or inquiry. Certain biologic processes and clinical behaviors actually resist the forces of complexity; despite immense perturbations, such as smoking, HIV exposure, or immense emotional stress, the human body often returns to a stubborn homeostasis. But for numerous other processes and behaviors, the effects of complexity apply far more widely than any of us are willing to admit. Minimally credible clinical and outcomes studies all factor in age, sex, race, co-morbidities, insurance status and smoking status, and adjust their conclusions accordingly. Acres of warehouses are stacked to the ceiling with commercial research data that aren't even minimally credible. In both realms, as countless studies of the same clinical and/or health care business phenomenon draw divergent conclusions, mystification tends to emerge as the rule, not the exception to that rule.

I have never seen nor heard of an outcomes study that factors in the variable of "patient stoicism." And yet the likelihood of patients' understating or overstating the severity of their physical symptoms may be the single most important determinant of how a heart attack or stroke is diagnosed, ruled out, or treated in an emergent setting. Although hundreds of studies have measured heart attack outcomes based on age, race, sex, surgical utilization patterns, and drug choices, one sticks out for its uncanny findings: a patient's rate of survival has less to do with the type of surgery he or she receives than it does with how far he or she lives from a hospital with a cardiac cath lab (McClellan, McNeil, and Newhouse, 1994). Where somebody decides to buy a new house or how vocal they are about their chest pain are indeed "small factors with large consequences." Joe Olson may have saved himself not by going back to the womb and correcting the way his aortic cells were dividing, but by crying out sixty-one years later, in earnest, for help.

RATIONAL IRRATIONALITY

Which returns us, unhappily, to our airplane drunk. As if the principles of complexity theory related to medicine were not enough to discourage our enthusiasms for ham-fisted clinical reengineering, yet another important element of complexity is let loose in the clinic: patient behavior. Much of what physicians can and cannot do is ultimately not in their control, but in the control of patients and their families, few of whom act "rationally" during a medical crisis. Even if physician clinical behavior could be analyzed and modeled fairly, the sheer irrationality woven into the experience of major disease or injury produces chaotic "perturbations" in every patient's medical action and reaction. Joe Olson's compulsion to smoke, despite heart disease, hypertension, and a postsurgical stroke, was his stoical way of medicating his depression and fear of death. It does not make sense to most of us, but it is what he did. By contrast, his wife with inoperative breast cancer may have begged for the physical torment of a bone marrow transplant that we now know to be futile, swallowed a garden of medicinal herbs, and overmedicated herself because of her own depression and fear of death. There is a rationality to her irrationality, borne of the most harrowing crisis a human being will ever face.

The implacability of this behavior is expressed with lyricism and poignancy by the old Arabian proverb: "He who has health has hope, and he who has hope has everything." Consistent with this most profound of human truths, seriously ill patients and their families are righteously indignant and endlessly demanding; faced with the specter of permanent disability or death, we all expect immediate access to every possible medical resource or life-saving measure, at any cost. The absence of this irrationality and desperation would, paradoxically, be a clinical indicator of depression. Viewed through this prism, we quickly see that this irrationality is quite reasonable—once again, a higher order of patterning borne of physiologic chaos. All the managed care twaddle about the economics of prevention and wellness aside, the biggest financial black hole in the U.S. health care system is the ICU. The MCOs would be better advised to focus all their energy and attention here and in the hospice—fully cognizant of and working in the context of medical and behavioral complexity that wracks both— rather than focus so much of their efforts on the relative nickels and dimes of routine care.

The same problem of a patient's irrationality afflicts those who feel and appear healthy, but are not. Patients are noncompliant with their physician's orders, they stop taking their medications for asymptomatic diseases, they lie to their doctors about their smoking and sexual practices, and then they demand state-of-the-art technology when the inevitable occurs. Most patients do not accept accountability for their medical choices, but do demand it from their caregivers. This is a learned behavior, reinforced over decades of generous public and private health insurance coverage and relatively untouched by recent attempts to ration that coverage through managed care instead of tearing down the whole system and starting over. Consistent with American consumer culture in general, as patients we want everything, are willing to pay for nothing (except alternative medicine, of all things), and resort to litigation when the worst consequences of our own behavior results in a bad medical or reimbursement outcome. How many years will it be before the drunk who had to be dragged off my airplane at LaGuardia demands a liver transplant, paid for by the rest of us?

Nature and its complexity rule our bodies, and medicine is engaged in an epic struggle against both. Lucky for us, our medical-miracle technologies and dedicated practitioners often win the battle, occasionally through high-drama heroics. Consider the experience of one patient who, according to press reports, was "gigantically pregnant with twins when she had a heart attack. In the hours that followed, she had open-heart surgery at the same time her twins were delivered seven weeks early by Caesarean section" (Stingl, 2000). Why did nature run amok for this patient? Because she forced it to. She had tried for five years to get pregnant, had visited "an army of infertility specialists," and finally conceived via artificial insemination. Delivering twins seven weeks early while undergoing major heart surgery may make for great television, but it is also a complete financial disaster for somebody. The informed observer cannot help but wonder how badly this case blew all annual financial projections for the patient's employer, health insurer, or at-risk medical providers. Such clinical travesties are the high-cost exceptions that greatly outspend the normal rules. We will always count on medical technology to help us contravene against nature. And when we are dying, most of us will fight to the bitter end.

In the vocabulary of complexity theory, irrational patients represent "friction" in a system that would work much better if only they did not act like patients. As Gleick describes it, "Without friction a simple linear equation expresses the amount of energy you need to accelerate a hockey puck. With friction the relationship gets complicated, because the amount of energy changes depending on how fast the puck is already moving. Nonlinearity means that the act of playing the game has a way of changing the rules" (Gleick, 1987, p. 24). The irrational demands that patients make of our health care and medical systems—from choosing cheap managed care coverage and then railing against limited access to care, to consuming vast quantities of fatty foods and then demanding obesity drugs—constitute major friction in the already complex equation of delivering medicine. Joe Olson's smoking represented significant friction, as did his noncompliance with his doctor's medication orders.

MISGUIDELINES

Taken together, all these elements of complexity explain why business strategies designed to impose clinical standards on physicians and hospitals do not work. The voracious appetite of managed care for medical care guidelines and measurement systems has driven it through countless fast food windows for "solutions" that are crude at best and dangerous at worst, failing as most do to account for the incredible complexity of medicine.

One of the most visible and controversial efforts in this arena has been the widespread distribution of hospital length-of-stay guidelines by the actuarial and consulting firm Milliman & Robertson (M&R). These well-intentioned formulas for how long a patient with a given diagnosis should remain in the hospital are, according to the firm, written by "highly experienced full-time doctors and nurses and represent a compilation of best practices drawn from medical literature, practice observation and the expert opinions of nationally recognized physicians" (Walker, 2000, p. 10). Unfortunately, the guidelines also have nothing to do with reality. Two studies that compared them to actual clinical experience, conducted by HCIA using the largest hospital database in the country, show that actual patient stays in even the most efficient and cost-effective hospitals in the United States—its "100 Top Hospitals"—greatly exceed the M&R length-of-stay guidelines. According to a report in *Managed Healthcare,* the two studies—one comparing M&R goals to the average of all pediatric patients nationwide, and the other comparing the benchmark lengths of stay of the hundred top hospitals—looked at "more than 3.5 million pediatric cases in 1998 in hospitals across the country. M&R's goal length for a hospital stay for a child with bacterial meningitis is three days, but the study says the U.S. average is 8.6 days and for the 100 Top Hospitals benchmark it is 8.3 days, both found in actual practice" (Walker, 2000, p. 12).

124

This is one among countless examples of our attempts to mold medical reality to health care's expectations. Most of those attempts fail, and all for the same reason: except for the most egregious lapses in clinical judgment, physicians and hospitals simply cannot be begged, economically coerced, or browbeaten into doing things differently than they ought to be done. National average length-of-stay data represent the aggregation of several million clinical dramas, exceptions, and uncontrollable factors. This phenomenon explains the accurate observation of many that although practice patterns may change with the imposition of external scrutiny, as soon as the scrutiny is removed, the patterns revert to where they started. In *Chaos*, Gleick describes this phenomenon as it pertains to physics. "You could add noise to this system, jiggle it, stir it up, interfere with its motion," he writes, "and then when everything settled down, the transients dying away like echoes in a canyon, the system would return to the same peculiar pattern of irregularity as before. It was locally unpredictable, globally stable" (Gleick, 1987, p. 48).

This describes to perfection the failure of managed care to attain any of its population health goals, as detailed in Chapter Three. The MCOs' constant shuffling and reshuffling of patients and physicians in the medical system have no lasting effect. People still go to see "their" doctor, demand the latest medical technologies, and make lifestyle choices that compromise their health. Managed care's obsessive number-crunching fails to account for the complexity of our entire health care system—and within the medical system couched inside that system—an aggregation of small factors at play in every individual encounter between caregiver and patient. Complexity theory, which centers on the truism that small factors determine the entire outcome, has rattled the world of science, challenging its century-old presumptions. As Gleick notes, in traditional science "there was always one small compromise, so small that working scientists usually forgot it was there, lurking in a corner of their philosophies like an unpaid bill" (Gleick, 1987, p. 14). In health care, those compromises are enormous. These unpaid bills—runaway health care costs and the growing number of uninsured people—are perfectly commensurate with the magnitude of the intellectual compromises embodied in managed care.

MY DATA CAN BEAT UP YOUR DATA

How big are these compromises? Businesses like HCIA and M&R got started because for years nobody in health care had a clue how to measure some of the most basic things. The health care industry is uniquely antiquated in its lack of empirical self-knowledge. We still do not know with any certainty something as simple as the average pay for physicians by specialty. Or which type of hospital provides more charity care, for-profits or not-for-profits. Or what the real medical loss ratio is for most MCOs. In health care, two answers to the same question, often using *nearly* identical data, never agree. Much larger versions of the rounding errors that triggered Lorenz's discovery of complexity theory flourish in studies of the U.S. health care system.

You are painfully aware of this problem if you read *Modern Healthcare* with any regularity. In 2000, the magazine published eight different sets of numbers drawn from surveys of physician pay. The *tightest* range in average compensation was reported for internal medicine: one survey claimed the figure to be $152,823, another put it at $116,000. The *broadest* reported range was even more amusing: the survey of surveys revealed that average compensation for oncologists could be as high as $321,067, or as low as $181,400, depending on which survey you believed. Even more tellingly, there was no consistent pattern among the specific surveys as to which reported higher figures and which reported lower ones across specialties. More chaos, more confusion, and a ridiculous variety of answers, depending on whom you ask and what you want to do with the data.

Also in 2000, *Modern Healthcare* reported findings from two studies of for-profit hospital charity care patterns, published in the then-current issue of *Health Affairs*. After not-for-profit hospitals convert to for-profit status, they spend less on care to the poor, according to one of the studies (Pauly and others, 2000). In the same issue, however, a second study questioned the level of community benefits not-for-profit hospitals provide in exchange for their tax-exempt status. The question of the impact of ownership conversions on community benefits is not easily answered, the article said with a palpable sigh. "It all depends on how you want to spin it," one commentator told *Modern Healthcare's* reporter. "The reality is it depends on what you measure" (Bellandi, 2000c, p. 8).

Indeed. Which is why attempts to legislate even the simplest standards in the clinic are not only problematic but highly politicized. In 2000, California passed a law that made it the first state in the country to mandate specific nurse-to-patient staffing ratios. "Many around the country, especially unions, are watching to see how California will handle implementation of the new law," reported *Modern Healthcare* (Lovern, 2000a, p. 3). How California pulls this off will be no mean feat. According to the article, the California Hospital Association and Association of California Nurse Leaders argue that the ratio should be one nurse for every ten patients; the nursing unions believe it should be one nurse for every four patients. The gaping six-patient-per-nurse difference is larger than the entire requirement as far as the hospitals are concerned. Not exactly a rounding error.

Finally, consider one of the most perplexing questions of all, the seemingly arbitrary answer to which informs and inflames perennial Congressional debate. When will the Medicare hospital trust fund go bankrupt? In the past three years, the number has swung from as soon as the year 2009 to as far off as 2026. Why? Because of the complex number of macroeconomic, medical economic, demographic, and epidemiological variables involved in predicting the fortunes of Medicare *next* year, let alone over the next decade. As a result, the specific bankruptcy year estimate published annually is hopelessly flawed, an exercise more in politics than meaningful prediction. HCFA calculates its estimates of future Medicare funding needs using linear modeling: the traditional spreadsheet, with its fixed interrelationships and static assumptions (Laster, 2001). In so doing, it makes no provisions for any "small factors"—like, say, the onset of a major new disease among the growing ranks of the elderly, or a technological breakthrough on a disease we already know about.

History teaches us how dangerous this analytic narrowness can be. Who could have predicted the costs associated with the strange new disease that emerged in the early 1980s, referred to at the time as "gay man's cancer?" By the mid-1980s, we understood the disease not as a disease but as a syndrome called AIDS. And we believed its contraction constituted a death sentence. Linear modeling by commercial and Medicaid actuaries helped us project both the incidence and the cost of palliating those death sentences. A few short years later (short, that is, unless you or someone you loved was dying from it), the drug industry started to tame AIDS with a handful of medicines, turning it into what may soon be a chronic, manageable condition. In the early 1980s, our confident presumptions about tuberculosis were just as wrong, unfortunately in the opposite direction. As we try to predict where health care and its costs will go in the next few years, how can we possibly predict where medicine will go?

FROM INFINITY BACK TO HERE

Medicine and health care are too complex for the engineering solutions we have been trying to foist on both systems for more than a decade. Put simply—and I say this after ten fruitful years in the health care information business—we cannot digitize many of the most important variables involved in our industry, nor predict their interplay, nor anticipate their effects on the rest of the system. Put even more simply, in the clinic, shit happens. Nobody can predict how, when, or why. If Joe Olson's doctors did not know this when they graduated from medical school, they certainly do now.

The rules of complexity theory rule much of what occurs in medicine and health care. These rules can barely be built into software that analyzes the behavior of simple economic markets. They *cannot* be built into software products or consulting processes for predicting and managing disease. Such products and processes all attempt to reduce the complexity of the modern medical encounter into simple sets of inputs and outputs. They try, clumsily and futilely, to fit Joe Olson's case into a spreadsheet.

Once again, Gleick's comments reveal the scope of our naivete. "Simple shapes are inhuman," he writes in *Chaos*. "They fail to resonate with the way nature organizes itself or with the way human perception sees the world. Almost no one in the classical era suspected the chaos that could lurk in dynamic systems, if non-linearity was given its due" (Gleick, 1987, p. 42). In our attempts to rationalize the delivery of medical care using lunkheaded managed care methods, misguided guidelines, and retrograde information technologies, we are thrashing around in our own classical period. We are getting nowhere, slowly.

We would have a prayer of breaking free from this conundrum if we embraced rather than denied the hard truth, working *with* the principles of complexity, when applicable, instead of in fruitless defiance of them. Where we start is with the same basic tenets of complexity theory that, by now, should be haunting you with its implications the way it has haunted me since Dr. Cook's e-mail in 1998. Yes, complexity theory as applied to medicine and health care is one more bugaboo we do not need in our busy professional lives. But it does offers us hope, and a set of practical solutions. As Gleick notes about fractals, "The degree of irregularity remains constant over different scales. Over and over again, the world displays a regular irregularity" (Gleick, 1987, p. 98). There is a path to this regular irregularity. It follows the trail already blazed by complexity theory's best students, and it parallels the application of complexity theory to disciplines outside of health care that have successfully understood its principles.

The essence of these applications is the management of expectations within broader, acceptable boundaries. Dr. Leonard Laster gives two excellent examples in a *Washington Post* article. Alan Greenspan and the Federal Reserve Board manage inflation using principles of complexity theory; they do not attempt to manage its daily wiggles but successfully keep it in a preset range. The Army Corps of Engineers manages floods through a series of levees high enough to keep water in place in rural areas during normal periods of high rain, but low enough so that those same levees will breach far upstream of major cities, thus minimizing the aggregate economic and human toll of a major flood. The health care version of these two examples is simple: we cannot tell doctors, hospitals, drug companies, and other providers what to do and expect them to fall into line, we can only create boundaries and manage against what is unacceptable beyond those boundaries. Joe Olson and his providers actually do fit into a spreadsheet, but only in a very large cell full of contingent functions.

Let us apply this expansive medical idea to a health care challenge. An organization cannot build a detailed health care business plan for the next five years and expect it actually to work. Anything but a five-thousand-page document would be too rife with "rounding" errors, too ignorant of the small events that can have big consequences. As Dr. Cook argued in that first e-mail, "Goals are more important than plans. Strategic planning in health care, in its current business school mindset, is worthless. One little thing, like HCFA's OASIS regulations for home health, can derail a complete set of plans without invalidating the goal of improved home care. Detailed plans greater than six months in scope usually break down" (John Cook III, e-mail to the author, Sept. 1998).

I will be the first to admit that this is indeed bitter medicine to swallow for all of us trained in and helping to perpetuate the business school mindset. It grates on all those who passionately believe that better information technology, statistical analysis, care guidelines, operations research methods, and more sophisticated financial and legal mechanisms will fix what is wrong with our health care system. Collectively, we have invested billions of hard dollars and working hours in businesses to mobilize all these things in the service of medicine. My own personal struggle with this may be summarized perfectly in a quote by Leo Tolstoy. "Most men, including those at ease with problems of the greatest complexity, can seldom accept even the simplest and most obvious truth if it be such as would oblige them to admit the falsity of conclusions which they have delighted in explaining to colleagues, which they have proudly taught to others, and which they have woven, thread by thread, into the fabric of their lives." Ouch.

Although Tolstoy's quote sounds like the resignation letter from a national MCO's medical director—finally admitting that all of his efforts resulted in the same outcomes for patients in an unmanaged system—it also offers a ray of hope. Once fully grasped, complexity theory is indeed a simple and obvious truth. At the same time, trying to apply its principles to the world around us is the most important and profound of all intellectual challenges we will ever face in our lives (with the exception, perhaps, of that pesky meaning-of-life thing). Confronted by the chaos that rules much of our health care and medical systems, do we collapse into nihilistic despair over the impossible complexity and unpredictability of these systems? Do we give up on ever being able to know what really destroyed Joe Olson? Or learn what his providers could have done differently? Or do we work fully and joyously within the context of complexity, accepting all of its limitations, perplexities, and great challenges?

Instead of trying to reengineer care, impose bogus rules on ourselves, and micromanage everything we do for patients, we need only to set boundaries on acceptable clinical behaviors and outcomes. We will end up with the same or better results. And in the process, we will waste far less of the money earmarked for people's medical care than we do today.

CHAPTER 6

Vaporware.com

Those of us actually building the Internet know that it allows inefficient processes to be inefficient on a scale previously unimaginable.

Archibald Warnock III,
astronomer and Internet entrepreneur

This week, using the Internet, I verified a dozen credit card transactions, found and purchased an out-of-print book, checked on the balance of my retirement account, tracked a FedEx package on its way to Chile, ordered a custom-built laptop computer from Dell, calculated various refinancing options for my mortgage, and booked a stay at a wilderness adventure lodge in Alaska. Elapsed time for all of these transactions: forty-nine minutes.

To refill a prescription for Claritin, an allergy drug I have been taking for five years, I had to call the pharmacy. They had to call my doctor, and my doctor had to call them back to authorize a new prescription. When I drove to the pharmacy, the prescription had not been filled. My health insurer recently started switching Claritin prescriptions to Zyrtec and the pharmacists thought it best to check with me before they called my doctor again to authorize the change or let me pay the extra for my doctor's orig-

This chapter was originally published by Project HOPE as "Vaporware: The Failed Promise of the Internet," in the November/December 2000 issue of *Health Affairs*. Copyright © 2000. www.healthaffairs.org.

inal drug choice. Elapsed time to refill one routine prescription: four and a half hours.

Since the advent of PC-based computing in the mid-1980s, successive generations of information technology (IT) have been promoted as the panacea for what ails the U.S. health care system. Better health care information systems, few would disagree, mean a better health care system: less fragmentation of medical delivery across geographic space and time, an infrastructure to identify and reduce variations in care, robust data sets to predict and manage costs more accurately, and the list goes on. Our pursuit of these goals as an industry has generated a long and wearying list of IT's boldest promises and most spectacular failures: the smart card, Community Health Information Networks (CHINs), telemedicine, the Electronic Medical Record (EMR), client-server "enterprisewide" systems, and in the mid-1990s, the clinical data warehouse (Starr, 1997; Kleinke, 1998c).

Then came the Internet, billed as nothing less than the next panacea for what ails the U.S. health care system. The health care Internet company presentations that have dominated the major health care investment conferences since the late 1990s are a colorful blur of PowerPoint graphics for products and services that for the most part do not exist, and probably never will. Suspend your disbelief, and you will quickly discover from these presentations that, because of the ubiquitousness of the Internet, health insurers are hungry to install Web-based systems that will allow them, finally, to process provider payments faster; physicians and hospitals will soon be readily sharing patient information; and patients with chronic diseases will be so well managed remotely by computer-savvy doctors that they will never again darken the doors of an emergency room.

Feel as if you have seen this movie before? I have, and I do not like the way it turns out. In the early 1990s, the largest hospital information systems vendor, HBO & Company (HBOC), went on an acquisitions binge, purchasing a far-flung constellation of niche vendors that provided the software running in the back offices of hospitals, physician practices, labs, and health plans. The company convinced Wall Street that demand for these products would continue to grow under a managed care–driven rationalization of the typical U.S. health care organization. HBOC further convinced Wall Street that these separate products, when controlled by one consolidating software vendor, could be successfully integrated, comarketed, and interoperated. Thus it positioned itself as the future Microsoft of a consolidating, integrating health care industry.

In 1998, HBOC sold itself to drug distributor McKesson a few short months before its sprawling business imploded, driving McKesson's stock from a historic high of $95 at the time of the acquisition to a fifty-two-week low of $19, before the damage was fully written off by Wall Street (King, 1999b). The company's fundamental problem was a disconnect between what works in a PowerPoint presentation and what works in a U.S. health care organization. In the same way that the predecessor vendors of smart cards, CHINs, EMRs, and so on, all failed, HBOC's strategy to interconnect health care organizations failed—not because its technologies did not work but rather because both its business growth plans and its IT product strategy collided with the labyrinthine complexity and economic conflicts that are inherent in today's health care system.

Is the Internet different? The largest player to emerge from the frenzy of health care Internet fantasies was WebMD, a company created from the merging of Internet start-ups WebMD, Healtheon, OnHealth, Medcast, and CareInsite, established software vendors and transaction-processing companies Actamed, Envoy, MedEAmerica, Kinetra, and Medical Manager, and equity stakes in nearly a dozen other companies. At the height of that frenzy in early 2000, Wall Street valued this colossus of high concept—complete with its three chief executives and three corporate headquarters in different regions of the United States—at $2.5 billion. This valuation was based on 1999 revenue of a scant $102 million, almost all of it derived from sales of non-Internet software and transaction-processing services acquired with WebMD's inflated stock.

WebMD's insane market valuation was driven by a steady parade of "strategic alliance" press releases, the sum total of which were more conflicting and self-contradictory than even the wildest rationalizations for HBOC's acquisitions in the mid-1990s. Like numerous other health care Internet companies that have raised huge sums of money based on ideas for products they might one day build and install, WebMD has been promising to use the Internet to connect all of health care's many constituencies: physicians, hospitals, labs, pharmacies, employers, health plans, and of course, patients. How the company would ever actually consummate this grandiose plan grew more problematic with each new press release. Throughout this chapter, which argues that the Internet's promises will inevitably collide with the U.S. health care system's realities, WebMD will be held out as an example of much of what has been attempted—and much of what will fail—in Web-enabling the U.S. health care system. At the height of the madness, WebMD represented 30 percent of all publicly traded investment capital in the health care segment of the Internet industry. For this reason, most health care IT companies for years were unable to raise investment capital without a WebMD strategy. WebMD also provided a perfect example of the term *vaporware.* Used by IT purchasers in the HMO, hospital, and physician group practice communities, vaporware may be defined best through this classic understatement made by a hospital CIO to a *Modern Healthcare* reporter, "The sales side and the deliverables side are not always identical."

Why the mismatch? Because WebMD and the other well-funded health care Internet companies with the same business plan have all been racing to create comprehensive connectivity among health care organizations that, unfortunately for those companies, are in competition for patients and dollars. For an example of the problems in attaining true connectivity across a health care system of competing organizations, we need look no further than WebMD's so-called strategic alliance announced in January 2000. According to a WebMD press release dated January 10, 2000, the company entered into a five-year deal with the CVS chain of drugstores for "exclusive" use of the its on-line pharmacy by physician and patient users of the WebMD Web sites. What did this mean for the 38.5 million Americans and Canadians whose pharmacy benefits were managed by Express Scripts, which requires its members to fulfill their on-line prescriptions through its own competing Web-based pharmacy? Or the 50 million Americans whose pharmacy benefits were managed by PCS, which is owned by Rite-Aid, archcompetitor to CVS, and whose members were required at the time to use

Drugstore.com for their on-line prescriptions? It meant that any physician group that accepted a free Web site from WebMD (funded by investor Microsoft) for the purpose of routing prescriptions electronically for all its patients had an onerous, paper-based administrative task made still more complex by its Internet provider, not less so.

Business deals like WebMD's exclusive agreement with CVS indicate that such Internet connectivity companies are even more confused or self-deluded than such pre-Internet IT connectivity companies as HBOC. By the end of 2000, as WebMD inevitably started to collapse under the weight of its own contradictions and broken promises, after successfully gobbling up some of the Web's best start-up companies, a sad fact about Web-enabling the U.S. health care system was emerging: the Internet would solve none of health care's underlying organizational problems while merely distracting its IT-hungry customers one more time with vaporware.

NIGHTMARE ON WALL STREET

The rapid rise and fall of the sprawling WebMD vaporware empire was symptomatic of a chronic problem on Wall Street: there is too much money chasing too few workable health care IT businesses. Since the 1980s, investment bankers have been arguing that because health care is the nation's largest and most information-intensive industry, it is on the verge—perpetually on the verge—of rapidly expanding its spending on IT. The health care information company where I worked in the 1990s, HCIA, raised a large sum of money through an initial public offering (IPO) in 1995, as did several other health information systems, products, and services companies. Much of the same investor enthusiasm that helped us all go public back then accompanied the rush of IPOs by health care Internet companies in the years since. Wall Street successfully took us all public by publishing research reports showing the chronic underspending of health care organizations on information systems and services.

Circa 1995, during the first health care IT gold rush, the conventional wisdom on Wall Street had it that managed care would compel all health care providers to invest in IT by finally making them accountable for their clinical operations and outcomes. (How providers would raise the money to purchase this IT, given managed care's primary task of reducing payments, was unclear.) In 1998, after most of the first class of health care IT companies had disappointed investors because of lackluster product sales, the conventional wisdom on Wall Street had it that Y2K would force health care organizations to spend more to replace, rather than fix, outdated IT systems (Kohn, Corrigan, and Donaldson, 2000). Two years later, a number of health care IT companies missed earnings targets because of a slowdown in sales that resulted from health care organizations spending their IT budgets on fixing, rather than replacing, outdated systems. A year after that, the conventional wisdom had it that the Institute of Medicine's (IOM) widely discussed report on ninety-eight thousand annual deaths resulting from medical errors would compel health care organizations to invest in IT that identifies and routs out such errors.

When Wall Street stock promoters are short on rallying events like managed care or the IOM report, they go back to arguing the same pristine piece of logic: because health care organizations have spent proportionately little of their operating budgets on IT, they simply must start spending more. At a conference in 2000, an investment banker told the audience to expect a "coming rash of IT spending by hospitals now that Y2K has passed" just a few months after *Modern Healthcare* released its annual purchasing survey showing that hospital spending on IT was holding constant that year at 2.6 percent of total operating budget—the exact same percent as in 1999 (Morrissey, 2000).

But bashing Wall Street for its self-serving self-deceptions is easy and not really fair. Like the rest of us, investment bankers are also health care consumers. They are responding to what we all witness every time we try to cope with our health plan on a payment matter, make an appointment with our doctor, admit a family member to a hospital, or simply try to refill a prescription: a cacophony of unintelligible processes, redundancy, and complexity. Health care is choking on its own paperwork. Doctors are not really computerized, hospitals and health plans are barely so, and customer service for the typical patient ranges from neglectful to abusive. Meanwhile, all else in our economy is moving toward ever greater levels of ease, automation, and convenience. The mess is so enormous and costly, there simply has to be a business opportunity—or so the thinking on Wall Street has always gone and continues to go with the recent funding of the health care Internet companies. As part of their IPO promotion, Healtheon, WebMD, and the other connectivity companies all sold themselves not on their tried and tested IT solutions but on health care's chronic IT problems. Since 1997, the IPO prospectus for every Web-based health care connectivity company (Healtheon, WebMD, xcare.net, Cybear, and so on) has begun with a lengthy description of the transaction-processing problems of health care, not the transaction-processing solutions offered by the vendor. This is akin to arguing that, because hurricanes are so destructive and costly, a new business to stop hurricanes simply has to work.

Such thinking grossly underestimates the scope, magnitude, and complexity of health care's IT problems, which in turn make those problems worse. They are made worse still when combined with Internet fever spread to health care. Judging from conversations with colleagues in the business and policy communities, the sudden faith that the Internet will fix health care's chronic IT problems seems also to have affected those who really should know better, those who understand how complicated health care is, how resistant to easy fixes, and how often its boldest IT promises have failed. Yes, the Internet makes it easy to find and purchase an obscure book, get a recommendation for and directions to a new restaurant in a foreign city, and share secrets about one's sexual fetishes with complete strangers. This does not mean that the Internet's underlying technologies, superior as they are over previous generations of IT, will be able to fix the U.S. health care system. Health care's fundamental problems are not IT-based problems; they are economic, legal, regulatory, organizational, and cultural problems.

If anything, by providing patients with instant, universal access to more medical knowledge and resources than they ever knew existed, the Internet is certain to *exacerbate* health care's fundamental problems, almost all of which stem from irrational consumer behavior, uneven patterns of utilization, and runaway costs. These are the problems that managed care was supposed to fix, which it attempted to do for the most part by adding still more paper-based processes specifically to constrain consumer demand, utilization, and costs. Taken to its extreme, one can argue that the *last* thing the U.S. health care system needs is the Internet.

A FIX FOR HEALTH CARE'S PERMANENT LOVE TRIANGLE?

Observers of all political stripes—myself included—have always argued that a fundamental source of health care's core dysfunctionality is the economic disconnection of purchaser from consumer, and both from producer. The third-party payment system (actually a fourth-, fifth-, sixth-, seventh-, and eighth-party payment system, as discussed earlier in this book) complicates even the simplest of transactions. Third-party insurers are surrogates used by government and corporate purchasers to police utilization and costs across the health care system; they are not in the business of paying quickly, for obvious, legitimate reasons and also because of less obvious, perverse economic incentives.

If an IT-based system that interconnects all health care constituencies were ever implemented, the third-party payer would have to drive the process. Unlike chronically fragmented providers, misfunded government agencies, and employers focused on their core businesses, third-party insurers have the critical mass, scale, and relatively easy access to funding needed to effect this interconnectivity. Insurers also have the closest thing to a connectivity mandate: they are already in the transaction-processing business. A central feature (and flaw) of the health care information business is the financial origin of most of the "medical" data underlying its products. Almost all databases eventually used to analyze medical utilization, costs, provider performance, and patterns of care started out as transaction databases for paying medical claims (Kleinke, 1998c).

Healtheon (now part of WebMD) has been trying to Web-enable the big national insurers since it started business in 1997. As of this writing four years later, the company is still struggling to do so. This may be seen in the company's dearth of new payer customer announcements and in the continued featuring in its advertising of the Beech Street PPO, the second payer for which Healtheon announced a demonstration project back in 1997.

140

Other connectivity companies have met the same fate: their press releases are chock-full of distribution agreements with each other but few have announced any major implementations of their technologies by national payer organizations.

If they would not buy, would they build? It was not until well into 2000 that six leading national insurers announced their own cooperative initiative—called Medunite—to build a shared Web-based system to attempt to accomplish what Healtheon has been attempting to accomplish for several years (Freudenheim, 2000). Another symptom of Internet fever, the Medunite announcement overcorrected the insurers' sluggishness to embrace the Internet with a grandiosity matched only by the ambitions of WebMD. It is highly unlikely that a coalition consisting of people from Aetna, Cigna, Wellpoint, Oxford, PacifiCare, and Foundation Health Systems will be able to schedule a meeting successfully, let alone plan, build, and implement anything that actually works. The insurers' track records on developing other IT standards has been horrendous, hence the need for standardization via legislation. (Such standardization was included in the HIPAA legislation back in 1996.)

The Internet has been a part of the public consciousness for several years. Why have the national insurers failed to embrace it through vendors like WebMD or actually created their own Web-based connectivity systems? There are two answers. First, insurers have embraced connectivity to the degree that they can. Second, they do not want to embrace connectivity to any greater degree for economic reasons endemic to the entire third-party payment system.

Contrary to what Internet entrepreneurs all argue in their investor presentations, enormous volumes of medical claims are already moving from providers to insurers electronically. As of 2000, 45 percent of all commercial claims were submitted electronically, 80 percent of all Blue Cross claims were submitted electronically, and 97 percent of all hospital claims were submitted to Medicare insurers electronically. These submissions occur through fast, reliable, secure private systems, many of which WebMD controls following its acquisition of three EDI "claims clearinghouse" companies. One of the goals of WebMD's business, if we are to read it literally, is to move these and the remaining claims submitted in paper form to the slower, less reliable, less secure public Internet. Why? Because the Internet will give patients and providers access to the progress of the adjudications of all those claims. For economic and organizational reasons, this is a losing proposition from the insurers' perspective, a concept we will explore momentarily. For now, let us assume that insurers actually did want to invest in an IT system that allowed patients and providers to track the adjudication of their claims, and thus be equipped to demand their reimbursements faster. Is this really possible?

Faster adjudication does not occur today on claims submitted electronically for the same reason that the thirty-day payment rules passed by numerous state legislatures in the late 1990s are ultimately toothless. Claims do not fail to clear insurers quickly because they are not submitted electronically. Instead, they fail to clear insurers quickly because the entire process of third-party payment presumes that every claim is potentially rife with errors and misrepresentations, and thus needs to be checked for a multitude of potential frauds and abuses. The thirty-day payment rules are all based on "clean" claims, a legal loophole through which insurers can drive the whole business. Fraud and abuse monitoring is still mostly a manual process because of the complexities and ambiguities of medical care. And given the sad fact that fraud and abuse policing has turned out to be HCFA's best idea in the past decade to "manage" the care it is purchasing for Medicare and Medicaid beneficiaries, it is safe to say that intensive fraud and abuse monitoring of claims will not go away any time soon. And this kind of policing may be the easy part. The adjudication of claims also involves mediating a series of complex and ambiguous medical codes against the mind-numbing number of variables associated with the nation's proliferation of health insurance benefit plans.

The people from Silicon Valley who thought health care was an easy Internet fix waiting to happen should have taken heed of earlier generations of IT companies new to health care. Those who started Healtheon (and WebMD) thought they saw in this enormous volume of claims paperwork an enormous business opportunity. (For an entertaining look at the combination of hubris and naivete about health care that was behind the founding of Healtheon, see Michael Lewis's highly readable book, *The New New Thing*, published in 2000.)

"Look how easy it is to use a VISA card to pay for goods and services around the globe," was the thinking among companies like First Data Corporation, which operated a massive credit card clearinghouse before venturing into health care. "Surely we can build a system like that to pay medical claims in our own town, right?"

Like the IT engineers working today at WebMD and the other health care Internet start-ups, what those established companies found was a bit more complicated than they expected. They discovered that clearing a typical insurance claim involves, for starters, the following queries:

- Is the patient a member of the plan?
- Is this particular service covered by the patient's benefits plan?
- Is there secondary insurance that should cover this service?
- Is this service related to an incident that may be attributable to (and therefore separately reimbursed as) a workers' comp, disability, or accident event?
- Is this service consistent with the patient's clinical diagnosis, history, age, and sex?
- Is the service, if covered, medically necessary?
- Has the service, if covered, been preauthorized?
- Is this submitting provider qualified to provide this service?
- Is the provider a member of the network?
- How much do we pay this particular provider for this particular service?
- Has the patient's deductible or major medical been met this year?
- Did the patient pay up front and are we reimbursing her . . . or the provider?

Not quite the same thing as clearing a VISA transaction, which involves the sum total of the following queries:

- Does the customer have enough credit on the card to cover the purchase?

- Has the card been reported as lost or stolen?

- Is this an authorized merchant?

Several dozen major corporations, including First Data Corporation, Equifax, CSC, and General Electric, entered the health care IT business in the early 1990s. They believed that automating the payment of claims was an extension of their core competency of automating financial transactions. They were wrong, and almost everyone of them exited the business, often with significant write-downs of the companies and other assets they acquired to enter it. What they discovered at the heart of claims adjudication was a computing, content, and analytic nightmare, not a missing telecommunications infrastructure. Once again, in health care connectivity is not the problem, complexity is. The Internet is ready-made to solve the first problem, not the second. This has been one of the hardest lessons for WebMD and the others to learn.

The health system complexities that have sullied the ambitions of today's health care Internet companies and yesterday's well-meaning corporations are a huge convenience for the health plans. These complexities obfuscate the larger barrier to insurers adopting a universally accessible Web-based system to speed up claims adjudication. In the insurance business, the "float" rules. The float is a pool of dollars generated by prepaid premium dollars the health insurer invests while *not* paying claims from it. If the process of claims adjudication is haunted by a computing, content, and analytic nightmare—*not* the insufficiency of the current telecommunications infrastructure—this nightmare is good business for health insurers that make money by sitting on money.

As the Internet connectivity companies like to point out, many of the queries included in the preceding list can be answered from disparate payer information systems via one of the Internet's most important technical advantages: open access to legacy databases. But open access is the last thing health insurers want to promote. If they did, they would have provided that open access—to eligibility, claims status, deductible amounts—through earlier generations of IT, including the electronic claims systems currently in use. But precisely the opposite works in the plans' economic favor. This is why they block on-line access to benefits eligibility, ask providers for clarification after a service is rendered, deny reimbursement to patients pending additional documentation, and switch prescriptions to "preferred" medications, forcing pharmacies, doctors, and patients into a four-hour game of phone tag for a simple refill. In the process, a large percentage of all paper-based transactions fall through the cracks, forcing everyone to start over again. This ghastly administrative inefficiency is the financial lifeblood of a health plan, when the premium dollars to pay those claims are earning 8 percent in corporate bonds. For a health insurer, the incremental administrative costs associated with managing a mess larger than it needs to be are trivial compared with the investment gains associated with *not* cleaning up that mess in the first place.

Indeed, this may be the U.S. health care system's dirtiest little secret. Health insurers do not make money by managing care, they make money by managing money. The health insurers could have fixed the adjudication problem over the Internet in the late 1990s, they could have fixed it with the CHINs in the early 1990s, and they could have fixed it with smart card technology in the 1980s. The persistence of the typical health insurer's perverse economic motives is one of the reasons why Healtheon, after trying to build a Web-based claims submission system for several years, finally surrendered and acquired legacy claims clearinghouse vendors instead. Unfortunately, the acquisition of three claims transactions companies (for example, Envoy) makes the job of turning the combined Healtheon-WebMD vaporware into functioning products even less likely. Such a conversion would require cannibalizing the only revenue stream the company has to report to Wall Street; it would also require it to force all those acquired programmers, engineers, customer service people, and so on, to abandon the proprietary information technologies they have been building and maintaining for decades.

Mindful of the economic and operational obstacles to bringing better IT to bear on the administration of health insurance, I found it personally exasperating to read *The New New Thing*. A description of Jim Clark's entrepreneurial journey from the founding of Silicon Graphics and Netscape to his creation of Healtheon, the book marvels at Clark's raucous, can-do spirit. With more amusement than skepticism, the author watches Clark throw tens of millions of his own dollars—and all his vision, energy, and previously unchallenged faith in IT—at the U.S. health care system (Lewis, 2000). Intentionally or not, *The New New Thing* illustrates Clark's gross underestimation of the magnitude and complexity of the health care system he was trying to fix with Healtheon with an endearing, if annoying, naivete that doomed him to fail.

If Jim Clark has spent his entire career ahead of the IT curve, then his statement in an April 2000 speech may be the best leading indicator of what will happen, in the end, to WebMD and the other vaporware.com companies. "There are a lot more efficient ways to put your money to work [than health care]," he conceded (*Silicon Alley Reporter*, 2000).

IS THERE A DOCTOR IN THE CORPORATION.COM?

What other efficiency, quality, and cost problems built into the traditional health care system is the Internet supposed to fix? Web-based connectivity is commonly promoted by health care Internet companies and their Wall Street backers as a belated solution for the fragmentation among physicians, physician groups, hospitals, hospital departments, other provider facilities, and ancillary services. If you believe the advertisements for some of the leading Internet companies—led again in boldness of promise by WebMD—then you believe that a common Web-based system will finally integrate medical delivery, allowing physicians and hospitals to resolve an economic and professional conflict that has existed since the emergence of the modern medical system in the 1890s.

Unfortunately, the obstacles to achieving this long-sought integration have nothing to do with IT and everything to do with the modern medical system. They range from the most obvious, tangible regulatory hurdles, like the anti-kickback and Stark self-referral laws that have foiled numerous efforts to integrate doctors and hospitals over the past ten years, to a large number of more subtle, but even still more intractable cultural problems deeply embedded in our system. To put it more bluntly, hospitals and physicians do not play well together; they never have and never will. A shared Internet initiative will not change that. Hospitals and physicians compete for large numbers of patients (for example, hospital outpatient versus office-based surgery), they function at economic odds for other patients (for example, Part A DRG-based payment compels hospitals to speed up the discharge of patients, whereas Part B line-item service payment compels physician specialists to slow them down), and they have a long, bitter history of failing to work together to accept economic risk for patient populations (for example, the failure of most PHOs and many IPA-based MSOs in the 1990s) ("PHOs Losing Steam," 1998).

As discussed in Chapter One of this book, the anti-kickback and Stark laws have complicated attempts by hospitals and physician groups to work together; trying to comply with these outdated, cynical laws has forced providers to create additional, often multiple corporate layers for the simple purpose of joint contracting with insurers for selected types of patients or populations. These laws have also fully precluded numerous attempts at economic alignment between hospitals and physicians, most recently the once-celebrated gain-sharing arrangements that would have rewarded physicians for helping hospitals manage inpatient costs more efficiently ("Gain-Sharing Illegal," 1999). Will these same laws affect the deployment of Internet-based systems across hospital and physician groups? They will if precedent is any guide. Both the Stark and anti-kickback laws have complicated—and in many cases fully precluded—the IT industry from building and installing software systems that connect physicians and hospitals. At HCIA we attempted to deploy several such systems in different ways for different purposes, but in all cases legal counsel advised clients that their deployment would invoke both the Stark and the anti-kickback laws. The easiest and most obvious application of a shared hospital–physician group Web site—integrated patient scheduling—flies directly in the face of these laws because the effort would be designed specifically to manage the flow of patient referrals.

The less obvious impediments to Web-based integration involve deeply ingrained economic distrust and cultural conflict between physicians and hospitals, the definitive history of which is catalogued in Paul Starr's landmark book *The Social Transformation of American Medicine* (1982). If there were no such conflicts, then the shared computing systems promised by the Internet would have been a fait accompli three computing generations ago. Telescoping well beyond shared Web sites for scheduling purposes, the Internet's more energetic promoters argue that the Internet represents a new generation of open computing technology that will finally allow patient information to be shared across legacy clinical and administrative IT systems. This is the exact same set of claims made about clinical data repositories in the late 1990s, EMRs in the middle 1990s, and client-server technology in the early 1990s. None of these technologies attained widespread market acceptance, hence the collapse of HBOC and the earlier generation of IT vendors (Kleinke, 1998c).

So, why this numbing succession of IT failures, when much of our economy embraces new generations of IT so readily? After controlling for all the other economic, legal, regulatory, and cultural barriers to IT adoption, only one explanation remains: the practice of medicine really is an art. It is too complex to be digitized; it involves elements of chaos theory that the typical IT vendor executive would be hard pressed to grasp intellectually, let alone incorporate into product design; and most importantly, it involves a level of accountability that no other class of professionals in our economy ever comes close to facing.

As many promoters of Web-based fixes for the health care system like to create clinical scenarios to illustrate the pervasiveness and power of the Internet, let us create one of our own. A fifty-four-year old man is transported to the emergency room with chest pain, shortness of breath, and generalized anxiety. He is conscious, mildly disoriented, has high blood pressure, and his EKG shows an irregular heartbeat. He has been treated at this hospital before, his physician admits most of his patients here, and his physician's group has a shared Web site for scheduling, billing, and on-line access to shared patient data. In short, the perfect case to illustrate the power of the Web for a local patient in a stable care environment.

The sales representative from the Internet vendor that wants to build that site demonstrates to the hospital's IT department and its chief of medical staff what happens next. The emergency room (ER) physician logs onto a bedside terminal connected to the hospital's intranet, which downloads the patient's medical history from the hospital's various inpatient and outpatient databases, the physician group practice database used by the patient's physician, and the database from the reference laboratory that group likes to use. The bedside browser application also searches the patient's PBM (pharmacy benefits management) database, which is now on-line and accessible via secure access for providers, and the ER is able to view the patient's prescription history for the past two years. The on-line search finds that the patient has diabetes, recorded as diagnoses by both his primary care physician and his endocrinologist, and confirmed by a prescription for metformin. The search finds no drug allergies, no history of heart disease, an ongoing prescription for loratidine, and no other drugs. Based on this information, the ER physician does not order additional blood work to screen for other medications and orders lab tests, which rule out a heart attack. Based on these results, she diagnoses a panic attack and orders intravenous alprazolam, an antianxiety medication, to stabilize the patient before discharge from the ER. She also submits an electronic prescription for paroxetine, an antidepressant approved for the treatment of panic disorder that increases serotonin levels in the brain; she tells the patient to take this as directed until a follow-up visit in one month. Thanks to the Web-based system, the prescription is waiting for the patient at the hospital's outpatient pharmacy when he is discharged from the ER.

Three days later, the patient is back in the ER complaining of abdominal cramps, nausea, restlessness, flushing, and diarrhea. He has a fever and the same generalized anxiety that prompted his first ER visit. A different ER physician is able to access the updated records via the hospital's intranet. He assumes his colleague simply missed a diagnosis for pancreatitis (easy to do, given the symptoms), admits the patient for observation, and orders IV antibiotics for the pancreatitis and meperidine for the pain, both standard treatments. The patient's symptoms get worse, his blood pressure skyrockets, his heart rate increases rapidly, he has a massive heart attack, and despite lengthy efforts at resuscitation, he dies.

The postmortem? The patient had serotonin syndrome, caused by excessive brain levels of serotonin. It turns out that the patient had been suffering from clinical depression, and had been taking sertraline to treat it. Sertraline, like paroxetine, also increases serotonin levels in the brain. Why was this information not found by the hospital's intranet during that first ER visit? Because two months earlier, the patient's primary care physician had referred him to a psychiatrist who was not part of the same multispecialty group; the in-network psychiatrists were unable to see new patients for several weeks. The out-of-network psychiatrist the patient saw was part of a group that had stopped sharing data with the hospital because it was embroiled in an anti-kickback investigation regarding discounted golf course fees. The sertraline prescription did not appear in the PBM database accessed by the hospital's intranet because the patient had filled it at a local pharmacy, using a paper prescription; the PBM rejected the claim because it had not given preauthorization for the drug. The patient did not push the issue with the PBM because he was embarrassed by the diagnosis of depression, and so he bore the cost of the prescription and the visits to the psychiatrist himself. If the first ER physician had known that the patient was already on one serotonin-increasing drug, she never would have prescribed paroxetine for the patient after discharge. If the second ER physician had known that the patient was taking two drugs of the same class, he would (or should) have recognized serotonin syndrome, which is diagnosed clinically rather than through blood work or other diagnostic testing, and he also would have known not to give the patient meperidine, which frequently exacerbates or precipitates serotonin syndrome itself.

The case described is not unusual, either clinically or administratively; and it does not represent a failure of IT. The specific technologies required to build the Internet-based clinical computing infrastructure described by the sales reps are perfectly feasible, as outlined in excellent detail in a *JAMA* article by Clement McDonald (1998). What caused this unfortunate chain of events, killed the patient, and will inevitably throw the hospital and its two ER physicians into a medical malpractice action is the perpetual clinical uncertainty that enshrouds all of medicine as practiced—and litigated—in the U.S. health care system. Once again, the culprit in this case is not an IT-based connectivity problem but rather a health system–based complexity problem.

As every practicing physician knows (or should know), when the survival of a human being is the so-called work product, an information system supporting that work that is not 100 percent reliable is 0 percent useful. This hard, unalterable fact has made building usable closed clinical IT systems extremely difficult; it will make building a usable clinical IT system—out of the slew of still-emerging open technologies collectively described as Internet-based computing—next to impossible. In medicine, myriad variables are at play that have always forced physicians, despite generations of new IT systems, to revert to paper charts, ask patients to bring their pills with them to appointments, and treat patients more conservatively than they would if they had full access to all pertinent patient information.

For years, IT executives have blamed physician resistance to computers as a major impediment to widespread IT adoption in health care. But the real impediment has been perpetuated by the IT executives themselves: in the training manuals and other documentation for every health care IT product, usually on the very first page, is the vendor's legal disclaimer for any negative clinical consequences that occur in association with that product.

WHOSE PREFERRED PROVIDER?

In one significant way, the Internet *is* different from previous generations of health care IT, and different enough as an IT phenomenon to alter, fundamentally, the economic future of health care in this country. The Internet is the first generation of health care IT to engage the same stakeholders who have driven the health care system to its current size and sprawl: 178 million consumers with insatiable medical demands and close to unlimited insurance coverage. (The 178 million is calculated as follows: the U.S. population of 280 million, less approximately 44 million uninsured, less approximately 40 million children under the age of eighteen, less 18 million adults covered by staff or group model HMOs with no out-of-network provisions.) The Internet gives patients equal, universal, and unlimited access to clinical information, comparative quality and cost data on providers, information on treatment alternatives, and each other. In the short run at least, this kind of access will change everything about the economics of the U.S. health care system for the worse.

Patient access to information on the Web will inexorably increase demand for alternative providers, new products, and more services. Consider the following three stories:

- *Consumer Reports* tells the story of a family whose newborn had "a rare congenital disease called osteopetrosis that required a bone-marrow transplant to save her life. 'I found most of the information I got on this disease from the Internet,'" the mother told the magazine. "'The doctors in St. Louis who treated my daughter had never seen a case of it before'" ("Finding Medical Help," 1997, p. 27).

- *The New York Times* reports on one woman's search for a fertility doctor in the United States while she was living in Bermuda; all local physicians had failed to diagnose her infertility. She found one, and successfully conceived and delivered (Fein, 1997).

- According to the same *New York Times* article, a woman who lives near San Antonio found a specialist in a Boston hospital "through the hospital's Web site when she was searching for help to learn why her 3-year old daughter, who has hearing problems, began losing the precious few verbal skills she had." The patient underwent a series of surgeries to correct a congenital defect in both ears and her hearing was partially restored (Fein, 1997).

A number of revealing themes are common to all three stories, typical of the popular media's coverage of patient use of the Internet. Each case uses an emotionally charged clinical situation to appeal to readers. Each associates a positive outcome with the self-empowerment embodied in the

patient's use of the Internet. Each involves a patient finding a treatment alternative well beyond the confines of his or her local medical delivery system. And each case represents the inducement of medical resources, a net increase in costs for the health care system.

Without the Internet, the patients in these three anecdotes would have been left to cope with a local medical system unable to help. With the Internet, the health insurers responsible for medical care for these patients now have additional bills to pay—or administrative costs to bear in their efforts to deny paying them.

Although patients with chronic diseases have always had a vested interest in researching their conditions and various treatment options, the Internet significantly accelerates, simplifies, and streamlines the process. Patients who previously were forced to comb through traditional libraries (an obvious barrier for those weakened or immobilized by disease) now have at-home access to global library resources. Thus, those most disabled by their diseases should experience, as a population, the greatest net gains in access, clinical self-education, and demand for leading-edge (that is, more expensive) drug therapies. This process of consumer empowerment will be encouraged by those with the strongest commercial interest to do so, ranging from the dozens of commercial consumer health care Web sites (for example, Mayo Oasis, Medscape, WebMD) to the drug companies who provide most of the advertising and other sponsorship revenues for such sites (Waldholz and Moore, 2000).

A riveting example of how this plays out on the Internet is the traditional publishing and Web presence of the living miracle Lance Armstrong, who won the grueling Tour de France bicycle race two years after being diagnosed with advanced testicular cancer, and then won it again a year later. Among the many heroes in his recent best-selling autobiography *It's Not About the Bike,* is the Internet and the access it gave him to information on his disease and alternative treatments for fighting it (Armstrong and Jenkins, 2000). Go to one of the patient-support Web sites associated with the Lance Armstrong Foundation—cycleofhope.org—and you will discover that it is sponsored by Bristol-Myers Squibb, manufacturer of four of the five chemotherapeutic drugs used to save Armstrong. Woe to the health insurer that tries to say no to a patient who finds out about and demands any of these drugs—regardless of what the insurer would rather pay for—when that patient is getting his daily inspiration from the living example, writings, and Internet presence of Lance Armstrong.

Along with the wealth of clinical information accessible by patients on the Internet is the large number of "e-communities" of fellow patients. Although the supporting technologies vary, the social structure of a patient e-community is essentially the same. A group of patients with the same disorder converse electronically about their disease, treatment experience, quality of providers, and other matters central to their medical struggles. Patients participate in these e-communities by posting comments to groups engaged in an ongoing, topic-specific electronic discussion, submitting articles or other resources to a common repository, and "chatting" in real time. They also subscribe to mailing lists, requesting that topical information be e-mailed to them as it becomes available, whether from a single, authoritative source or from other members of the mailing list itself (Bennehum, 1998). At this writing, the Internet hosted more than ninety thousand list groups and more than thirty thousand newsgroups. Traditional medical literature confirms the existence of clinical, educational, and psychological advantages associated with a patient's ability to communicate with other patients with the same affliction (Devine, 1996; Baker, 1996). Despite their well-documented wariness regarding patients' retrieval of medical information on the Web, even physicians endorse the use of on-line support groups by their patients (Miller and Reents, 1998). As a result, there is not an existing illness that does not have its own Web site and e-community. The pervasiveness of e-communities is evident across the epidemiologic spectrum: at this writing, there are more than 500 Web sites and more than 570,000 Web pages associated with diabetes; even more tellingly, there are 9,705 Web pages associated with Huntington's disease.

As many have observed, some of the clinical information on the Internet is excellent, some questionable, and some downright dangerous. (One of the most important jobs of the primary care physician in a Web-enabled health care system will involve helping patients differentiate good information from bad.) Because of the wealth of information about diseases,

154

patients with access to the Web will be equipped, often erroneously, to advocate strongly for medical interventions that their physicians may recognize as inappropriate because of differential diagnoses or other mitigating clinical circumstances. The physician who holds his or her ground may end up losing these patients to other physicians willing to provide that intervention. Conversely, certain patients may challenge their physicians on the side of caution; they may be disproportionately influenced by rare adverse events associated with the disease and its recommended treatment as the result of access to clinical information or Web-based exchanges with other patients. One of the reasons why physicians express the greatest skepticism if not outright hostility to patient access to clinical information on the Web is a patient's inability to interpret such information. They argue that patients will jump to erroneous conclusions about the severity of their conditions, arrive at faulty self-diagnoses, or latch onto symptomology to corroborate their hypochondria (Miller and Reents, 1998).

The sum total of all this information access will be increased demand for medical resources, many of which the demanding patients would never have known existed. Although it is too early to test this hypothesis with controlled populations, it can be inferred from the source in the health care system that provides most of the actual spending on health care Internet services. Most of the revenues for today's health care Internet companies derive directly or indirectly from the pharmaceutical industry. The drug companies have spent lavishly on traditional direct-to-consumer (DTC) advertising over the past five years, and the continued increase in their spending on TV and print ads indicates that it pays off. Such spending has coincided almost perfectly with increases during the same time period in aggregate pharmacy *cost* inflation, defined as prices multiplied by utilization, an important distinction from the supposed price inflation claimed by opportunists in the managed care and legislative arenas (Dubois and others, 1998).

The Internet is the DTC movement in overdrive. Web-based DTC allows drug companies to target specific patients with specific diseases; it does the same thing for Web-savvy hospitals and other providers who are seeking to attract patients for their more profitable service lines. The goal of both types of Web-based DTC is patient pull-through, a business strategy designed to neutralize the utilization and cost control goals of today's health insurers. According to a *Wall Street Journal* report, more aggressive use of the Internet for DTC drug marketing and distribution is one of the explicit goals of the recent $75.7 billion merger of GlaxoWellcome and SmithKline Beecham into the largest global pharmaceutical company (Waldholz and Moore, 2000).

What happens when you combine Web-based DTC by drug companies and providers with hundreds of thousands of independent Web sites and communities? You get the biggest run on the health insurance bank in the history of the industry. As health plans have learned over the past few years, when access to new treatments is withheld from consumers, they will use the courts, and their legislators, to break down managed care's controls. The first wave of this consumer sentiment crested with the development and overwhelming popularity of point-of-service plans and the dissolution of small, closed networks. The tidal wave of consumer preference for choice and access comes in the form of the universalized provider "network" represented by the Internet. When fully swamped, the nation's health insurers will be what Jeff Goldsmith refers to, in a *Health Affairs* analysis of the likely effects of the Internet on the entire health care system, as "virtualized." Goldsmith argues that "consumers are bypassing both the health care delivery and the health insurance system and seeking the information they need to frame their transactions with both systems" (Goldsmith, 2000). Indeed, consumers are asserting the ultimate, inevitable primacy of their demands via the Internet while continuing to assert in the courts and labor markets that their bills must be paid by someone else.

What eventually comes to define a "preferred provider" in a Web-enabled health care system will change inalterably as patients use the Web to find what *they* perceive to be better providers. To examine the full effects of this, we need to revisit for a moment some of the more absurd, if often-repeated rhetoric of managed care: employers claim to want to steer employees to the best health plans and health plans claim to want to steer those same employees to the best providers. In reality, both want to steer patients to the cheapest plans and providers. If employers really did want to steer their employees to the best plans, then more than 12 percent of them would require NCQA accreditation in selecting their health plans—and more than 1 percent of employers would make the NCQA's HEDIS data available to their employees to support their selection of individual health plans (Gabel, Hunt, and Hurst, 1998). A study reported in *JAMA* found the same disconnect between what people in health care say and what they actually do. There is a strong pattern indicating that health plans steer patients to hospitals that have both lower prices and inferior performance measures on quality (Erickson and others, 1999). The failure of employers to use HEDIS to help employees select better health plans—and the health plans' preference for "unpreferred" providers—are perfect examples of what Carl Schramm, former executive director of the Health Insurance Association of America, refers to as "the health care rhetoric gap" (Carl Schramm, personal conversation with the author, 1997).

The Internet is in the process, finally, of filling in this health care rhetoric gap by providing consumer information about health plan and provider quality. The Internet in general has gained such popularity because it allows people to combine numerous criteria for a search and comb through enormous lists of sources for specific data—book titles by author, local movies by zip code, airfares by price—and then directs them to precisely the information they need. Hospital and physician data are no different, just more complicated to develop into objective and fair information. The Internet provides the first feasible way of transforming large data sets into provider and health plan performance information for consumer use. A number of Web businesses have emerged to do precisely this, ranging from niche Web start-ups like HealthGrades.com, which is seeking to become the *Consumer Reports* of provider performance on the Web, to large established health portals like The Health Network, a heavily trafficked site that publishes the Mercury Awards, a scoring of hospitals by market and service line, to several independent Internet content companies acquired by WebMD.

These Internet companies are doing what employers and health insurers should have been doing all along but did not for economic reasons—and what pre-Internet health information businesses like HCIA and

Medstat could not do for technical reasons. The provider performance information being published by the Internet content companies is built from public data sets compiled by the HCFA, the NCQA, state hospital associations, and others, and used by insurers for their own selection of providers. (While at HCIA, I observed that insurers default to public data sets because of the insufficient size, currency, or reliability of their own claims databases, a fact that we successfully commercialized through medical informatics systems built for numerous national managed care organizations.) Such data sets have always been available to the public, but because of their size were not mobilized for consumers until the Internet. These same data sets fostered the growth of pre-Internet health care information companies like HCIA, which used them to develop and market products to hospitals, health plans, drug companies, and other businesses. These business-to-business information products were restricted to institutional users because it was impossible, before the Web, to deliver focused, user-friendly information to consumers who need specific bits of information, not entire information systems. At HCIA, we struggled through most of the 1990s to come up with a business model under which we could develop and market our large, clinically rich hospital databases for consumer use. In those pre-Internet days, we were unable to find one, as were all of our competitors.

What is the result of consumers using the Internet to get information on higher-quality health insurers and providers? Once again, the answer is higher medical costs. As patients finally get access to everything from Web-distributed HEDIS data to hospital performance scores, they will flock to the higher-quality insurers and providers, not only driving up costs in general but emboldening those same insurers and providers to raise their prices. (As already discussed in this book, a central feature of the health care rhetoric gap created by managed care is the belief that higher-quality and lower-cost providers can exist, over time, in a market economy.) Many have argued that patients using the Web to find providers will finally bring price sensitivity to health care consumption, and a number of emerging Web businesses are based on this principle. The exact opposite is more likely to occur. The retail purchase of a major medical product or service like a cardiac bypass surgery assumes a rational consumer at a time of extreme personal crisis. In fact, people will never seek the lowest bidder when it comes to their own physical and emotional well-being; indeed, they will actively seek out and select the highest bidder, presuming (usually correctly) that higher cost connotes higher quality, just as in the rest of our economy.

Such behavior will continue to be encouraged by the moral hazard underlying third-party payment of medical care. American medical consumers will always demand the best, and they will always expect it to be paid for with somebody else's money. If you believe that defined contribution health funding will fix this—at this writing, the twaddle du jour among numerous pundits—you need look no further than the marketplace failure of MSAs or the legislative fate of health marts as surrogates for peoples' unwillingness to bear financial responsibility for their own medical decisions.

OPEN YOUR E-MAIL AND SAY "AH"

A corollary argument popular among health care Internet companies and their backers is that even if the Internet does induce demand for more medical resources, the associated costs will be offset by various types of remote doctoring that the Internet will soon enable. Such remote doctoring falls into two categories: formalized e-mail-type physician "visits" by patients, and disease management systems that route patient clinical measurements from their home computers or medical devices to centralized nursing stations. If we believe that either of these new services will displace, rather than add new costs to the health care system, we should look at the realities of medical practice and the sad fate of telemedicine over the past decade.

Many have argued that e-visits between physicians and patients have the potential to preclude some office visits entirely. The key issue associated with the supplanting of office visits by e-mail is not privacy, as many have argued. As recently as 1997, fear of electronic theft of credit card numbers was expected to be a major barricade to consumer purchase of goods over the Internet. Rather, the key issue is bound up in the culture of medical practice: it involves the real reasons that people want to "see" their doctor, and the real reasons why doctors still insist on "seeing" patients when—long before the Internet reached critical mass—they could just as easily consult over the telephone.

Granted, my view tends toward economic determinism, but I always thought that doctors saw patients to make money. A strong impediment to e-visits with physicians is the same one that blocked the widespread acceptance of telemedicine: reimbursement. Because telemedicine represented a significant improvement in access and quality of care for patients in remote locations, it also represented induced costs for their insurers. With telemedicine, patients can "see" leading specialists without onerous all-day drives across rural landscapes; without telemedicine, those same patients either make the drives, delay the encounter until they can, or forego the service altogether. Small wonder HCFA and the health insurers have not rushed to figure out a way to regulate and pay for the bulk of telemedicine services.

By contrast, HCFA and the managed care industry might be happy to figure out a way to reimburse e-visits; unlike telemedicine, e-visits may prove to *reduce* total costs. This, of course, is exactly why physicians, then, will *not* embrace them as alternatives. Until reimbursement to physicians for providing an e-visit is worked out, they will continue to regard such alternatives warily, as yet another threat to their income. This same impression of e-mail is the reason physicians most often cite for their reluctance to enter into e-mail communications with patients (Miller and Reents, 1998; Goldsmith, 2000). (This problem is already solved for patients covered by the disappearing reimbursement method of capitation, of course; an e-visit that preempts an office visit supplants a cost rather than revenue opportunity for the physician.) Will e-visits—even if adequately reimbursed and thus embraced by physicians—displace office visits demanded by patients? Or will they merely become one more service to be delivered and reimbursed by insurers? This leads us into one of the Internet's biggest health care challenges: if e-visits do add new services and costs, insurers will not want to pay for them; if they supplant old services and reduce costs, physicians will not deliver them. This same exact conundrum will extend to the Web-based remote monitoring systems, which are really e-visits of another variety. If this extra IT-driven service adds costs, then insurers will not pay;

if it displaces physician visits, then physicians will not authorize its use with patients for whom they retain ultimate liability.

In addition to these obvious economic issues, important clinical realities jeopardize the feasibility of both types of remote visits, whether e-mail-based or monitoring system–based. There are no well-designed studies confirming this, but dozens of primary care physicians have told me in private conversations that 25 to 35 percent of their office visits involve people who are not really sick, but lonely. This is particularly true, they report, among the elderly and disabled populations, many of whom regard a doctor visit as the central event of their day. E-mail and remote monitoring will not only fail to displace these visits but will greatly increase the means and thus the frequency with which these same patients "access" the health care system out of loneliness and lack of anything else to do that day.

Finally, the biggest clinical obstacle of all to remote doctoring is a central feature of medicine that the entire IT world has forgotten in its twenty-year rush to digitize the health care system: a large part of the practice of medicine is nonverbal, visual, tactile, and intuitive. An entire career spent designing health care IT systems was put into painful perspective during one argument I witnessed recently in the doctors' lounge of a busy Denver teaching hospital. The exchange embodied the totality of our struggles to rationalize health care through better information systems.

Two physicians on the hospital's faculty were arguing heatedly over whether to proceed with an expensive diagnostic surgical procedure for a patient. When a third physician walked in, the two presented a unified set of facts to her, including a long list of lab values and other clinical details, and asked her opinion. The third physician, a highly respected and published clinician and researcher replied, "I don't know. I'd have to see the patient."

NIGHTMARE ON WALL STREET: THE REMAKE

If there is more money than workable business ideas on Wall Street, then the health care Internet sector embodies this problem at warp speed. Despite all the administrative, political, cultural, and clinical realities described in this chapter—and despite the ultimately unhappy history of earlier generations of health care IT companies—vendors continue to receive funding, regardless of the tenuousness of their business plans. Despite the bursting of the Internet bubble in 2000, several dozen companies still managed to raise collectively tens of millions of venture capital and IPO dollars based on their intentions to create systems that may one day be used by patients and physicians to e-mail each other. If anything, the investment community's hunger to fund what will ultimately prove to be vaporware grows only more acute with each successive generation of IT failures.

What is particularly noteworthy about the Internet generation of health care vaporware, however, has been a breathtaking acceleration of the inevitable. The same funding cycle through which the earlier generation of health care IT companies passed—accompanied by many years of operating real businesses—has affected the health care Internet companies in short order. This cycle, typical of numerous high growth sectors in the economy, involves the raising of highly speculative venture capital to fund new companies and launch products; the emergence of small, profitable businesses and the sale of their stock to the public to accelerate their growth and profitability; the acquisition of smaller niche players by an emerging leader, which becomes a larger, even more profitable company as a result; and the eventual sale, fire-sale consolidation, or asset liquidation of the remaining companies after slowed growth, missed earnings targets, and collapsing share prices.

As discussed at the beginning of this chapter, HBOC led the health care IT sector through this cycle before selling itself to McKesson and then crashing (King, 1999b). On a smaller scale, HCIA went through the same process, several years after crashing in the stock market, recovering, and merging with the Sachs Group. Medstat went through a hybrid version of both business resolutions, twice, at different points in time. In every case, the health care IT company built up a strong and admirable business, acquired other companies to fill out its product line, and inevitably ran into the limits of the demand for, and workability of, a burgeoning portfolio of health care IT products.

WebMD and several other companies skipped the first step. In less than two years, they went from start-up business idea to consolidator of other start-up business ideas. WebMD has also managed to relive another key chapter, in compressed form, of the sad history of HBOC: it uses creative accounting to boost its reported revenues and thus keep a strong, if empty wind in its investment sails. Although WebMD reports revenues from the legacy, non-Web-based claims processing companies it has acquired, its only actual Internet revenues have consisted for the most part of distribution arrangements with other Internet start-ups. Under these arrangements, the start-up obtained cash from WebMD in the form of an equity investment, and then returned that same money, often in a deal announced in the same press release, to WebMD for distribution of its products through the WebMD Web site. A typical example of such a deal involves SimplyHealth.com, an Internet start-up that agreed to pay $30 million in revenue to equity investor WebMD for distribution of its on-line health insurance brokering service, according to a WebMD press release dated June 2, 2000. At the time of this announcement, the service the company was paying WebMD $30 million to distribute had yet to become functional in any state except Georgia.

The P. T. Barnums running many of today's health care Internet companies would be good for comic relief if their actions were not ultimately so destructive. They have created tremendous cynicism about the Internet in the health care community. As WebMD and others burn through investors' cash to buy up other noncompanies and issue press releases instead of building real products, IT executives at health plans and provider organizations across the country grow ever more contemptuous toward what could have been the first truly revolutionary computing platform to come along since client-server in the mid-1990s.

Besides all the squandered investment capital, this is the real, if intangible cost we pay for the continuing proliferation of vaporware in the U.S. health care system. With focus, discipline, and patience, Internet technologies could fix *some* of the things that are wrong with health care in this country. But as long as its loudest promoters continue to sell the Internet as snake oil to fix everything that is wrong with health care, it has less and less of a chance of fixing anything.

CHAPTER 7

A "System" for
the Uninsured

D r. Peter Agnello is a third-year emergency medicine resident at University Hospital, a large teaching hospital in a western city. He chose emergency medicine for the same reasons he excelled as captain of his high school basketball team: he is good at leading motivated groups of people, and he relishes the adrenaline rush of making split-second decisions amid constantly changing circumstances and great pressure. He also values his free time and plays several sports, and he wanted a career in medicine defined by shiftwork, not paperwork.

Today in the hospital's ER, Dr. Agnello saw fifteen patients, nine of whom have no public or private health insurance. Five of the six insured patients constituted true emergencies: an older man with acute chest pain, a young man with a knife wound, a construction worker with a pneumothorax who had fallen from a crane, a child with suspected bacterial meningitis, and a woman suffering a large hematoma spreading out from her temple who insisted she had fallen down her basement stairs. The sixth insured patient had a bad cold and wanted antibiotics.

Five of the nine patients without insurance were emergencies by the time Dr. Agnello saw them, but all could have been prevented: a child with asthma on the verge of suffocation who had not been on any asthma medication for several months, a middle-aged woman with a runaway pneumonia that had set in several weeks earlier, an unmedicated multiple sclerosis patient in the midst of an acute attack, a schizophrenic patient who may or may not have been medicated, and a Mexican national ineligible for routine dialysis who, every week, Dr. Agnello or another resident admitted to the hospital for a three-day stay and "emergent" dialysis.

The other four uninsured patients were not emergencies at all: two had minor infections and needed antibiotics, one needed more of the diabetes medication she had gotten in the ER last month, and one was a fidgety young woman who reported excruciating back pain and knew exactly which narcotic would take care of it.

Dr. Agnello crumpled onto the threadbare couch in the residents' lounge, weary from a twelve-hour noisy blur of patients, nurses, and telephone calls. He would miss basketball practice again. Instead, he would spend the next several hours in the lounge, reviewing the day's cases with one of the ER's attending physicians, completing fifteen patient charts, filling out admission forms, and writing up the same explanation to the hospital's accounting department for the emergent dialysis admission.

Contrary to popular belief, we *do* have a health care system for the uninsured. They get their medical care in the nation's ERs, through a patchwork of poorly funded community health clinics, via hospitals' "charity care" budgets, from overworked medical residents like Peter Agnello, through pro bono care provided by physicians in their "free" time, and through drug giveaway programs sponsored by the nation's pharmaceutical companies. Like the rest of our health care system's architecture, this (non)system for the uninsured has been designed piecemeal and by accident, creating in the process the least efficient, most costly way to deliver care to a large segment of the U.S. population.

It's a vicious cycle. One of the largest drivers of unaffordable health insurance premiums and still more uninsured people are high medical costs. These costs are continually driven up because of the boneheaded way in which we care for the uninsured, who cannot afford those premiums in the first place. Three days' worth of "emergent" inpatient dialysis costs seven times as much as routine dialysis, a cost borne by all of us in several ways: supplemental Medicare payments to University Hospital, government funding of residency training for Dr. Agnello and his colleagues, lost tax revenues the hospital does not pay because of the tax-free status associated with providing such care, and the higher prices University Hospital charges to all its insured patients.

As discussed in Chapter Four, a sizable chunk of health care spending is determined not by patient demand but by provider supply. Much of this excess supply is the result of the growing number of medical residents, like Peter Agnello, which in turn is the result of funding for teaching hospitals like University Hospital, which in turn is the result of the legal and social mandate of U.S. hospitals to care for the uninsured. As Dr. Fitzhugh Mullan observes in the *New England Journal of Medicine,* "The number of residents has been determined by the staffing needs of hospitals, the availability of trainees, and public funding of graduate medical education. Even New York hospitals that committed themselves to reducing the number of residency positions under a special Medicare demonstration program have been reverting to their previous training patterns" (Mullan, 2000, p. 213). Why is this happening in New York? Because 27 percent of the city's residents have no health insurance, and nearly 75 percent of the care delivered in its ERs is for nonemergent or primary care treatable conditions (Billings, Parikh, and Mijanovich, 2000a, b). New York's situation stems from the large proportion of teaching hospitals across the city and is aggravated further by the conflicting missions of all such hospitals in a health care system funded by both public and private means.

In addition to the artificially high number of medical residents that pushes physician supply and health care costs past a true market equilibrium, there are other burdens for hospitals created by their conflicting missions and charity care mandates. These burdens are by necessity passed along by the hospitals in what they charge for insured patients. Health insurers translate these higher charges into higher premiums, after adding their own administrative surcharges, which the market then translates into more uninsured people. This vicious cycle explains why the percentage of working-age Americans without health insurance grew from 15.1 percent in 1979 to 23.3 percent in 1995 (Kronick and Gilmer, 1999). It also explains how the number of uninsured Americans actually grew during the late

1990s to 44 million despite the unchecked economic expansion and full "natural" employment of those years. So much for the effectiveness of the employer-based health insurance system enshrined in our tax code.

The Twaddle Echo Factor often tries to diminish the financial and economic pain of 44 million uninsured Americans by pointing out that many of them are young, healthy, and part of an insurable workforce. True. But it is equally true, in literal numeric terms, that many others without insurance are *not* young, healthy, and steadily employed. Such twaddle represents a gross abdication of the problem, it is intellectually lazy, and as too many of Dr. Agnello's medical cases illustrate, it is highly impractical. Even the youngest and healthiest uninsured people will get sick or injured at some point, and all of them will show up in the emergency room. In its study of the care delivered to the uninsured in New York, the *Commonwealth Fund* notes that "individuals who cannot afford the cost of an office visit, or who are unwilling to wait for care in overcrowded and understaffed community clinics or hospital outpatient departments, rely on emergency rooms for primary care" (Billings, Parikh, and Mijanovich, 2000b, p. 1). This explains why half of all visits to ERs across the United States are for nonurgent care like sore throats ("Second-Class Medicine," 2000). The Commonwealth Fund study found that, "excluding ED patients who were admitted to the hospital, three-quarters of all ED visits to New York hospitals in 1998 were for conditions that were either non-emergent (41 percent) or emergent but treatable in a primary care setting (34 percent)" (Billings, Parikh, and Mijanovich, 2000a, p. 2). The biggest travesty? "Seven percent of visits that required care in the emergency room were potentially preventable."

This is the hard reality of our nonsystem for the uninsured. They receive their care in the dumbest possible way, after their illnesses progress to the point of crisis. In the aggregate, all the unmedicated asthmatics, diabetics, schizophrenics, and patients with runaway pneumonia—treated by thousands of Dr. Agnellos in ERs across the United States—represent not only medical misfortunes but economic disasters, for us and for them. In addition to bearing the burden of a runaway illness, the uninsured patient's inability or unwillingness to buy health coverage carries a second punishment, one that often lasts longer than the illness itself. Many are forced into bankruptcy or have their credit ratings destroyed by providers seeking to collect payment for their services. For too many uninsured patients, a hospital's legal mandate to provide charity care is consummated only retroactively, after its efforts at collection—some of them ferocious and all of them practiced by both for-profit and not-for-profit hospitals—fail. For many, the so-called charity care budget is really a bad debt budget, dressed up for state and federal tax auditors. The horrors of this situation percolate in U.S. bankruptcy data: of the 1.2 million American families who filed for bankruptcy in 1999, 500,000 reported medical problems. According to *Consumer Reports,* more than 300,000 of them identified an illness or injury as the reason for filing ("Second-Class Medicine," 2000).

In addition, using University Hospital's emergency room for their primary care guarantees uninsured patients the poorest possible continuity of care. The same *Consumer Reports* article notes that "a person in the midst of a seizure gets treatment for the seizure but no investigation to determine the cause. A child in the middle of an asthma attack may be treated with medicine that opens the air passages but won't get medications to prevent future attacks. In the emergency room, uninsured diabetics receive treatment only when their blood sugar has climbed so high or sunk so low that their life is in danger" ("Second-Class Medicine," 2000). The ramifications of this problem showed up in a comprehensive study of primary care and preventive medicine patterns published in *JAMA* in 2000. The study found that uninsured adults were far more likely not to have had a routine checkup over the two-year study period; their "deficits in cancer screening, cardiovascular risk reduction, and diabetes care were most pronounced among long-term-uninsured adults"; and they were "less likely to receive potentially life-saving preventive care such as cholesterol screenings" and mammograms (Ayanian and others, 2000, p. 2061).

This may be exactly how we as a society want it, at a collective unconscious level that manifests itself in public policy and government funding choices. As discussed in Chapter Three, more generous primary care and prevention across a population does not pay off. This may be especially true if half the uninsured are indeed younger and healthier. Providing more proactive charity care in the community would be far more expensive than the "we'll see you in the ER when you're really sick" system we have today. This may be a cheaper proposition than providing the full range of health benefits for those too poor to afford insurance but too "well-off" to qualify for Medicaid. Our unconscious preference for this choice and the resulting nonsystem used to care for the uninsured is a national disgrace, considering our national wealth.

This preference is expressed in the way our government currently handles care for those without insurance. According to Havighurst, "Even though the notion of compulsory charity is an oxymoron, the nation has apparently adopted a policy of relying on hospitals' widespread ability and willingness to cross-subsidize uncompensated care for the uninsured as a principal safety net for those who fall through the gaping cracks of private coverage" (2000, p. 102). Much of the patchwork quilt that makes up our nonsystem for taking care of the uninsured is held together by one federal law, the Emergency Medical Treatment and Active Labor Act of 1986 (EMTALA). Havighurst notes that the law "requires hospitals participating in Medicare to provide their usual emergency screening to any patient appearing in the emergency room (not just Medicare beneficiaries) and to stabilize any emergency medical condition discovered—all without regard to a patient's ability to pay" (p. 102). This federal mandate, ironically, means that the uninsured in those states without mandated any-ER-access insurance benefits actually have *better* access to the emergency rooms than many insured people with managed care coverage. Go figure.

Through EMTALA, the federal government forces hospitals to provide generous primary care in their emergency rooms. Much of the paperwork that Dr. Agnello fills out at the end of the day flows from the various compliance rituals associated with this law. But besides this one law and its far-reaching effects, we have not established a clear, workable corporate tax accounting system under which hospitals can provide EMTALA-mandated care and still conduct business in the highly competitive private insurance market. Instead, the federal government puts yet more patches on the quilt: it provides supplemental payments of numerous types under Medicare and

Medicaid at highly politicized rates, and it prospectively "reimburses" for that primary care through graduate medical education funding, which subsidizes charity care in an oblique, and thus monstrously inefficient, way.

A NOT-FOR-PROFIT HOSPITAL BY ANY OTHER NAME

The government also attempts to subsidize charity care through poorly codified provisions in the tax code. Most hospitals are putatively nonprofit, even though most data reveal profit margins among the not-for-profits that are on par with their for-profit competitors. A not-for-profit hospital's tax-free status is threatened only when its charity care provision dips to such low levels that it sets off alarm bells at state or federal regulatory agencies or among consumer advocacy organizations. As with so much else in the health care system, the absence of clear, unambiguous standards forces the government to default to arbitrary enforcement—a reactive process that in turn encourages hospitals to game the system, fiddle with the numbers, and ultimately skimp on charity care. The rules of this game have generated that extra paperwork for Dr. Agnello to fill out for University Hospital's accounting department. This is not the hospital's fault; it is simply playing by a stupid set of rules. And while the government imposes and enforces arbitrary rules from the left, private market forces squeeze University Hospital from the right. Most hospitals may be not-for-profit institutions with sizable public missions, but nonetheless the competitive marketplace forces them to compete on price with one another and with the for-profits, thus motivating them financially to minimize their actual charity care. This explains why most (but not all) studies show that the not-for-profit hospitals rarely provide significantly higher levels of charity care than the for-profits do, and that profits earned by the not-for-profits usually exceed their charity care provision (Pauly and others, 2000; Reinhardt, 2000).

How do we fix this? We commit the entire hospital industry, which provides the bulk of medical care to the uninsured, to one clear direction. The combination of charity care mandates and market forces has divided every institution like University Hospital against itself and pushed the entire hospital industry into a competitive race to the bottom. A more sensible approach would be to choose once and for all an unambiguous tax-status path, rationalizing the process of hospital charity care through one of two very different, major, uniform changes to the tax code: we convert all hospitals to for-profit status and use the new taxes we collect to fund government reimbursements directly (or even better, to fund health insurance premiums) for the uninsured, or we convert all hospitals to nonprofit status and mandate uniform levels of charity care as a percentage of total collected revenues. A commitment to either option would be better than our current marketplace and organizational schizophrenia. Either option would encourage hospitals to provide medical services to the uninsured in a more proactive way, either one would do away with the hospital industry charity care endgame once and for all, and either one would be better than the worst-of-all-possible-worlds that characterizes today's health system for the uninsured. My recommendation would be the less intrusive of the two, converting all hospitals to not-for-profit status (because most already are) and mandating a level of charity care as a percentage of revenue. Doing this would avoid the complexities associated with taxation and redistribution of hospital profits. It would also reinforce normal marketplace effects as a not-for-profit hospital's increasing business success translated directly into more charity care. Ambitious graduate students and professional foundation grant-chasers take note: this proposal would be fascinating to explore, "score" financially, and formulate.

A different version of the same solution can be worked out for physicians, with more aggressive tax credits going to those practices that want to provide more pro bono services to the uninsured. Despite the business pressures created by managed care, many physicians remain philosophically inclined to care for the poor, even if the economics of their own practices discourage it. As they pass through residency training, U.S. physicians like Dr. Agnello develop their clinical skills while caring for the uninsured in teaching hospitals, enshrining charity care in the culture of medicine. As Dr. Bob Cutillo writes in *JAMA*, "The poor have always been at the center of the history of medicine as a healing profession and the future of the profession likewise will be inextricably linked with the critical issue of how we will care for the poor in our country" (Cutillo, 2000, p. 197). *Consumer*

Reports notes that "the realities of professional practice supplant this compulsion. Health-care providers that in the past have cared for the uninsured in part with leftover money from insured patients have seen those funds squeezed by managed-care cost cutting" ("Second-Class Medicine," 2000). A uniform tax *credit* for providing care to the uninsured—as opposed to its current tax deductibility—would start to reverse this insidious process. Determining how this would work, what it would cost, and how it would benefit the uninsured would be another fascinating, important avenue of inquiry for ambitious researchers.

Our current nonsystem for taking care of the uninsured through hospital charity care budgets and pro bono physician services is subsidized further by the nation's drug companies. As of this writing, fifty different pharmaceutical companies sponsor drug giveaway programs for the uninsured, resulting in the distribution of free drugs to 1.5 million people per year (personal communication, Jeff Truett, spokesperson, Pharmaceutical Research and Manufacturers of America, Jan. 2001). This is a noble effort, but it is a pittance compared to the need, a cup of water thrown on the desert. Unlike the charity care provided by hospitals and doctors, which consists mostly of unbillable medical labor, the drug company subsidies do not represent significant marginal costs to be subsumed by the system and cross-subsidized by those who have insurance. As a result, drug giveaway programs are a real bargain for society: the raw ingredient costs of free drugs are trivial compared to a drug company's R&D costs, which are fully reflected in prices charged to insured patients. Consistent with why the drug companies are the most profitable segment of the health care system, the leverage of medical technology—unlike the leverage of medical services—can have a disproportionately large benefit for the uninsured for low marginal cost.

Drug company programs that help the uninsured are commendable and important, and they represent the privatization of a social welfare program sponsored by those with ample resources to do so. But like every other piece of the patchwork quilt that is our nonsystem for the uninsured, the results are less than fully successful. According to the Kaiser Family Foundation's Commission on Medicaid and the Uninsured, "Thirty percent of those without health insurance don't fill their prescriptions, because of the cost" ("Second-Class Medicine," 2000). A third important avenue for exploration would be finding a way—again, probably using the corporate tax code—to expand the drug company giveaway programs from token gestures into meaningful contributions. Such efforts would be especially effective if conducted in tandem with the hospital and physician charity care-related tax code reforms suggested earlier.

If the drug companies rose to the occasion created by this reform, they could consummate the expansion of their giveaway programs by doing more of what they do best: actively promoting their uninsured patient programs to physicians. The drug companies already have big plans for promoting their products to Dr. Agnello when he finishes residency. Why not supplement this promotion with a few words about how they can help his most unfortunate patients? These efforts would be greatly rewarded in improved physician and public relations for an industry whose pricing policies and profitability have rankled the nation for years.

WAITING FOR GODOT'S REFORM PLAN

While we wait for these or other meaningful reforms, our nonsystem for the uninsured grinds on. Peter Agnello will finish his residency and another new doctor will take his place, University Hospital and its accountants will bob along on the ebb and flow of government funding, the costs of treating the uninsured will rise and be passed along to insurers, premiums will rise, and more people will lose insurance coverage. In the meantime, the patchwork quilt of charity care will grow ever more threadbare and the vicious cycle will spiral onward.

Without systemic reform, we will continue to suffer from a woefully incomplete public policy on provider-based charity care. Current government spending stems the worst bleeding but does not cure the problem. As of this writing, the federal government was funding three thousand community health clinics to the tune of $1 billion per year, with a measly $94 million increase—or less than 1 percent, a significant decline in real terms—earmarked for 2002. These clinics, along with the nation's ERs, are the cornerstones in a shadow medical system operating across the United States. "In storefront walk-ups, church basements, and community and day-care centers, clinics set up shop to provide primary care for the uninsured, often asking doctors to donate their time," according to *Consumer Reports*. "They pull together exam tables and boxes of medicine samples doctors have discarded, and they decorate the walls with colorful posters telegraphing information about vaccines and breast exams" ("Second-Class Medicine," 2000).

What is the quality of care like in this shadow medical care system? According to Dr. Fitzhugh Mullan, a physician who treats the uninsured at the Upper Cardozo Health Center in the District of Columbia, it is "primitive, irregular, unpredictable, and uneven." This unevenness was quantified in a study of physician treatment patterns published in *Medical Care* in 1996. "Physicians who were presented scenarios with insured patients recommended service for 72% of patients, and physicians who were presented scenarios with uninsured patients recommended the same services for 67% of patients" (Mort, 1996, p. 783). Most of the clinical ramifications of these findings may be benign. If so, then these data serve only to underscore the central problem with third-party health insurance payments—namely, the availability of coverage stimulates demand for medically marginal medical services. Would that this represented the entirety of the case. But other clinical ramifications of the gap in insurance-related treatment patterns can be, quite literally, malignant and lethal. According to a study in the *New England Journal of Medicine*, four to seven years after an initial diagnosis of breast cancer, uninsured women are 49 percent more likely to die than women with insurance.

Even as the uninsured flood the nation's ERs and overwhelm doctors-in-training like Peter Agnello, they are still getting substandard medical care. Our nonsystem of caring for the uninsured operates on an entirely different level than our system for everybody with private or public health care coverage. This explains the difference in Dr. Agnello's case mix: most of the patients he treated today with private or public coverage had truly emergent, nonpreventable conditions; most of those without coverage had just the opposite.

Dr. Agnello's patient mix sits at the tail end of our political and cultural choices. It is the most insidious outgrowth of our essential faith that the marketplace can best fund and deliver all our medical needs. We should be ashamed of this faith. In 1984, Ronald Reagan's speechwriters borrowed a quote from a colonial writer who characterized America as a "shining city upon a hill" for the rest of the world. Yes, we are, as evidenced by Dr. Agnello's admission of the Mexican national to University Hospital for dialysis every week. In Mexico, she probably would have died a horrible death ten years ago. Among our many blessings as a nation, most of us have instant access to the best that medicine has to offer. But as Mario Cuomo observed in a speech at the 1984 Democratic National Convention, "It is a tale of two cities." The uninsured hover around the edges of a system built and run for the insured, they dip in only when they get seriously ill, and this greatly complicates the functioning of the entire system.

If, as it appears, the spirit of Reagan has come to dominate the American political soul—if we believe that self-interest is the only interest, good medical care is an earned privilege rather than a human right, and the marketplace is the only way to deliver that care—then we need to use market forces to fix this disaster. There is only one way to do that: *make health insurance more affordable*. This is the spirit and substance of the health care reform plan proposed in the next chapter.

CHAPTER 8

A Simple Plan

Any damn fool can be complicated.
Woody Guthrie

I t is November 2008, open enrollment season for selecting health insurance coverage. Mary O'Reilly, a single mother of two teenage boys, is sitting at her home computer, selecting her health plan for 2009.

Mary works for a small company that used to buy fully insured coverage, subject to state benefits mandates and regulations. Because it did not have the financial wherewithal to self-insure under ERISA, the company nearly stopped providing coverage altogether when premiums soared in the late 1990s. Now Mary's company simply sets aside the money it used to pay for each employee's insurance and lets its employees pick whatever health plan they want.

Mary goes to a commercial Web service, enters her zip code, and a moment later is comparing the prices of three dozen different health insurers offering coverage in her town. One is a locally owned HMO, another a locally owned PPO. The rest are national HMOs, PPOs, and other kinds of insurers; their only offices are located in Connecticut, the Midwest, and California. One insurer is headquartered in Boston and conducts all its business over the Internet. The three dozen insurers all offer the same benefits package, but for different prices. If Mary chooses a plan that costs more than what her company has set aside, the difference comes out of her paycheck before taxes. If she chooses a plan that costs less, the untaxed balance accumulates in her medical spending account, which she can draw on for medical expenses not covered by the plan.

Mary picks the insurer in the middle of the pricing pack because a friend at church told her that it pays for whatever pediatrician and pediatric specialists its members want for their children. According to information on the independent Web site, the plan she picks also does not try to switch any of the drugs that a doctor prescribes. These are important things for Mary because one of her sons has diabetes.

Mary also likes the fact that this insurer spends 96 percent of her premium dollars on medical care, versus only 93 percent for the average insurer listed on the Web site. The accountants in Mary's company also like this aspect of the health insurer's offering. Back in the 1990s, the two insurers that the company had selected for their employees spent between 76 and 82 percent of the company's premiums on medical care. Because of the compounding effects of the wide differences in medical loss ratios, Mary's health insurance in 2009, on an inflation-adjusted basis, will cost 28 percent less than it did ten years earlier.

Mary hits the "submit" button, and a moment later her one-page policy for 2009—referencing the standard benefits plan and her monthly premium—appears on her computer screen.

Forget your politics. For better or worse, the "free" market will remain our nation's choice for funding health insurance and delivering medical care. Our only hope of fixing the health care system's biggest problems is to enact simple legislative reforms designed with one purpose: to allow the market to provide health insurance more efficiently and affordably. This is a significant and somewhat painful conclusion for the same author who wrote a book as recently as 1998 arguing that managed care would compel the market to reform itself. Contrary to everything I believed, argued for, and tried to help build a few short years ago, managed care has proven to be a complete, self-contradictory failure for Mary, her employer, her providers, and her son with diabetes.

In this chapter, I propose a three-point plan that will greatly streamline and simplify the ability of the health care marketplace to finance and deliver medical care. Each component of the plan incorporates three principles that have proven sacrosanct in the health care community, reflected either in market forces or stated public policy goals: consumer choice, continuity of care, and affordability of premiums. At the tail end of the marketplace chaos that managed care created in the 1990s, Mary is tired of playing shell games with the two insurers her company has been using. She wants simplicity, reasonably priced health insurance, and no barriers to medical care.

For there to be true health care consumer choice, we must reinvent one very important, far-reaching element of the U.S. health care system: we need to get employers out of the health care business. The continuing imposition of employers into the system reduces choice, interrupts continuity of care, creates mistrust, and adds numerous layers of costly, suffocating complexity to a system that is gasping for air. Only 50 percent of Americans with employer-based coverage have any choice of health plans, and only one-third can choose from among more than two plans (Kaiser Family Foundation, 1996). The situation is even worse for small companies: 91 percent of all firms with between 3 and 199 workers offer their employees a choice of just one plan (Kaiser Family Foundation, 2000). Employer restrictions on choice of health plans have created a self-defeating paradox: millions of Marys have demanded that MCOs erode the one thing that best characterized their original function and that serves as a requirement for their broader population health goals—the ability to select and deselect providers based on cost and quality. Nonetheless, the remnants of selection and deselection persist, at least in contracting and reimbursement mechanisms. This has forced Mary to switch her son's doctors, if only on paper, every time her company switches insurers. Once again, the current system provides us with the worst of all possible worlds: the narrowing of consumer choice by employers to a degree just sufficient to preclude real continuity of care both within and among health plans.

Continuity of care is critical, and it is the reason why employees seek always to overrun each new "care network" border almost as quickly as it is established. According to a study in *Health Services Research*, "Compared to the continuously insured, those insured but with a recent time uninsured were at high risk of going without needed care and of having problems paying medical bills. This group was two to three times as likely as those with continuous coverage to report access problems. Policy reforms are needed to maintain continuous insurance coverage. Currently uninsured and unstably insured adults are both at high risk" (Schoen and DesRoches, 2000, pp. 187–188). This makes economic as well as clinical sense. As Safran and colleagues note in *JAMA,* "From the perspective of resource use, an ongoing patient-clinician relationship is commonly understood to be most efficient. The medical and health services literature points to numerous and diverse ways that patient-clinician continuity can translate to cost savings" (Safran, Tarlov, and Rogers, 1994, p. 1584).

Finally, affordability. Most of the 44 million uninsured people in this country remain that way for one simple reason: health insurance is too expensive. Fully one-third of those 44 million people have access to insurance through their jobs or through the job of a family member but do not enroll because of cost ("Second-Class Medicine," 2000). A similar statistic is provided by an exhaustive study by the Employee Benefits Research Institute (EBRI) on employer-based coverage: 27 percent of surveyed employers report that "their employees decline dependent coverage because they cannot afford the premiums" (Fronstin and Helman, 2000, p. 15). The study found that 50 percent of employers who currently do not offer coverage would do so if the cost fell 10 percent and that nearly 70 percent of employers not offering health benefits cite high cost as a major or minor reason for not doing so. Who are the employees most affected by this affordability problem? Those who work for small employers like Mary's company. According to the EBRI study, "Of the 44 million Americans who do not have health insurance coverage, 36 million are in a family with a worker, and small firms employ 60 percent of uninsured workers. Since the vast majority of large employers offer health benefits, but many small employers do not, small businesses are the most crucial element in efforts to expand health insurance coverage in the current health insurance system and reduce the growing number of uninsured Americans" (Fronstin and Helman, 2000, p. 20). Because small employers are most likely to limit their employees' choice of health insurers when they *do* buy coverage, reforms that would

180

make all health insurance more affordable should be coupled with those seeking to neutralize the employer's role in the entire process.

Central to the three goals of choice, continuity, and affordability is massive simplification of the entire health insurance system. Such simplification cannot occur in health insurance markets broken up by state lines, characterized by regulation for one third of the market by the federal government and two thirds by the states, and offering its customers a seemingly infinite number of benefit plan designs. Our cues for simplification come from, of all unlikely places, the Medicare program. This is indeed a mouthful from someone who has articulated in excruciating detail—in forums ranging from the *Wall Street Journal* to dozens of health care conferences—the myriad problems with the current Medicare program. Yes, Medicare's reimbursement rules are a Byzantine nightmare for providers. Yes, the system is antiquated and unintegrated across care settings. Yes, the methods used to determine rates are highly politicized rituals. And yes, the reimbursement rules and rates are enforced through arbitrary and often vicious tactics. A plan for truly reforming the essential architecture and functioning of Medicare is long overdue, and would fill another book. But despite its many obvious problems, through its sheer stability and size the Medicare program has tremendous economic and administrative advantages that can be applied to all of health insurance. These advantages stem from one fundamental feature of the Medicare program: a generally uniform set of benefits. Providers may game the system and be punished mercilessly for it (just as they do under private insurance). But for the most part, most providers know what is covered and what is not, and so do Medicare's claims administrators. Medicare is a truly interstate program, regulated only by the federal government; it is completely portable for its beneficiaries; and aside from its often arbitrary dictating of artificial prices, it does not interfere in the provider-patient relationship, except in cases of gross provider misconduct. As a result, Medicare currently spends 98 cents of every funded dollar on medical care (Uwe Reinhardt, personal communication, Jan. 2001). Compare this to the 80 cents that a commercial health plan spends on medical care, and the source for the entire system's correction stares you in the face.

If we were to convert the entire commercial health insurance system to a uniform health benefits design, do away with self-defeating state-by-state regulation, and provide all consumers with access to those benefits either directly or through their employers on a tax-neutral basis, then the health insurance market would enjoy most of the economies of scale and other efficiencies of the Medicare program. We would suddenly "find" nearly 18 cents of every commercial health care dollar in free money. This 18-cent pickup on every dollar still allows for health insurance company profits; contrary to public opinion, insurers earn those profits outside this enormous administrative surcharge, mostly from investment income on escrowed premiums. As described in earlier chapters, health insurers make money by managing money, not by managing care. Applying this percentage to the $302 billion that employers spent on health care in 1998 would generate a windfall of $54.4 billion per year—the equivalent of $1,236 per uninsured American—more than enough for each to buy catastrophic coverage. To hold current medical spending levels constant under such a market liberation, the only truly necessary adjustment to this 18 cents would be the cost to insurers of continuing to provide utilization review, which Medicare does not currently do. If United Healthcare's expense item for this is credible, and as the second largest insurer in the United States, we have every reason to believe it is, then we would need to pull only 0.3 cents back from this 18-cent windfall (Benko, 2000). The remaining 17.7 cents of the health insurance premium dollar currently going to waste are spent on three things: coping with state-by-state regulation of health plans, administering a growing proliferation of benefit plan designs, and paying out commissions—four cents' worth on average—for health insurance brokers who feed on the administrative cacophony created by state-level regulation and their own endless benefit plan tinkering. These three features of the current health insurance system sit squarely in the crosshairs of this chapter's reform proposal.

Before pulling the trigger and outlining those reforms, I need to make two important points: first, I will gleefully defy the instinct of health system reformers to create entire new infrastructures to implement their reforms and thus consume in new administrative costs the very money they would free up. The compulsion of reformers to fix what is already too complicated by introducing a barrage of new "fixing" entities is what doomed the Jackson Hole Group's managed competition model. It made a laughingstock of the Clinton plan, which wrapped still more administrative packaging around the Jackson Hole Group's work. And it is characteristic of numerous other well-meaning reform proposals that are sound in principle but then get bogged down in heavy-handed implementation. A good example of this problem is the otherwise laudable plan that the AMA outlined in 1999 (Dickey and McMenamin, 1999).

I do not believe the cure for bureaucratic paralysis throughout the health care system is more bureaucracy. I remain a believer, with much qualification, in the marketplace as the best way to distribute goods and services, including medical ones. But I also believe that the U.S. health care marketplace needs to be liberated from its essential failures, most of which are the result not of natural market forces but of the distortions and intrusions of a series of accidental tax and regulatory policies. If stupid legislation got us into this mess, then smart legislation will get us out of it. Such legislation should seek to correct tax-code problems, simplify health insurance regulation, and develop standards that streamline marketplace processes. Beyond that, we can and should let consumers and health insurers do the heavy lifting of repricing and redistribution. With three dozen insurers competing for Mary's premiums—instead of the two now competing for her company's premiums—the price-performance ratio that drives real consumer markets will finally be brought to bear on health insurance.

My second point before we get started is more problematical. The elegance, simplicity, and feasibility of the reform plan proposed here represent an enormous threat to powerful economic forces and political interests. The plan will be fiercely opposed by those who make fortunes (or at least good livings) and create jobs by draining cash from the complexity of our current health care system—and by those who wield enormous regulatory power presiding over that complexity. The 18 cents of every health care dollar that I target as waste also happen to feed hundreds of thousands of hungry brokers, consultants, lawyers, accountants, vendors, government bureaucrats, and workers at all levels of the MCOs. Many will claim to care about Mary and her boys, but the shrillness of their opposition will betray their real interests. They will not go away without a nasty fight.

MY TAX BREAK IS YOUR TAX BREAK

An employer-based health insurance system, enshrined by tax advantages not bestowed on retail insurance consumers, is not only needlessly complex and inefficient but also fundamentally unfair. All things being equal, if Mary's company were to stop buying her coverage today, she would need to earn a dollar in pretax income to purchase what her employer is now getting for 75 cents. The result is a highly regressive tax system.

This explains why, according to a study reported in *Health Affairs,* 68.7 percent of de facto tax breaks—income in the form of health benefits exempt from taxes—granted in 1998 were for families with incomes of $50,000 or more per year; such families represent only about 36 percent of the population (Sheils and Hogan, 1999). In a separate study reported in *Health Affairs,* Havighurst notes that "a tax subsidy of this kind is insidious precisely because, in addition to being an off-budget public expenditure (amounting to about $125 billion in 1998), it can misallocate huge amounts of society's resources, yet be almost entirely invisible and painless at the level of individual producers, consumers, and taxpayers" (Havighurst, 2000, p. 88).

Many observers believe this inequity and its related misallocation of resources can be corrected by removing rather than expanding the tax exemption for health benefits. This may be a philosophically sound response, and it is one way to take employers out of the equation, but it is politically unfeasible. It also conflicts with American society's clear desire to promote public health, reflected in the exemption of certain types of food from sales taxes but not others. Nearly the same goals can be attained through public policy that extends, rather than removes, the tax deductibility of health insurance premiums—and deductibility for expenditures on legitimate, noninsured medical services—to consumers. The extension of tax deductibility to consumers for all medical expenses will eliminate the historic, tax-based incentive for Mary's company to provide and micromanage health benefits for Mary and her boys.

184

Under this reform proposal, referred to for the rest of this chapter as *tax parity*, employers can continue to provide those benefits the way they do now. Or they can provide an equivalent lump sum of tax-free funds to their employees—as Mary's company will do in 2009—to purchase their own care, in whatever mix of insurance and out-of-pocket services they desire, from whatever health insurer they choose. This second option rides piggyback on the popularity of employee flexible spending accounts that pay, in tax-free dollars, for deductibles and medical services that are not covered; it also mirrors the slow but inexorable movement toward defined contribution that is now standard among employer-based retirement funding (for example, 401k plans), and has been suggested by many as a way to liberate the health insurance market. It also takes advantages of the best features of the once celebrated Medical Savings Accounts (MSA), which failed to catch fire among employers specifically because of the complexity of managing them around the tax problem. Coupled with the universal plan design included in this reform proposal, the defined contribution effect flowing out of tax parity merely streamlines people's access to their health insurer of choice. The prices for these insurers will then stabilize along a marketplace continuum based on cost and perceived quality, just as they did for Mary when she sat down at her computer to make her own choices. Just like a real market.

With a standardized plan design and the consumer mobility created by tax parity, health insurance customers like Mary are free to choose whatever insurer they want: the one with the best customer service, the one with the fewest utilization review hurdles, the one with the most heartwarming TV ads. Mary's money, her medical care, her choice. The consumer behavior consequences of this tax code reform would mirror one of the goals of the AMA's reform plan, with its own proposal of tax parity. According to Nancy Dickey, the AMA's president, "The choice of health plan would be the patient's, not the employer's. We believe that many persons would be more sensitive to deficiencies in quality than their employers are; hence, health plans would lose enrollees quickly if they were unresponsive to individual patients' concerns about quality" (Dickey and McMenamin, 1999, p. 1307). Many of the specific features of the AMA's reform proposal would fold nicely into a system of tax parity. For example, "two-income families would be able to combine the separate employers' contributions in paying for their chosen health plan" (p. 1307).

Unfortunately, the AMA plan quickly goes astray. "Our proposal would require the establishment of a new set of organizations, Voluntary Choice Cooperatives (VCCs), to enhance patients' choices. By combining large numbers of persons in a common market, VCCs could both increase the number of health-plan choices and drive down the price of individual coverage toward rates that are currently available only to large group purchasers. Furthermore, the ability to choose a health plan through a VCC would be available to all persons, whether they were employed, self-employed or unemployed" (Dickey and McMenamin, 1999, p. 1307). With millions of Marys all shopping for a uniform benefit plan from among a dozen health insurers competing in their market—based only on price and perceived quality—the creation of this new type of third party would be unnecessary. In fact, as Mary's case illustrates, we already have that third party: the Internet.

Legislated tax parity represents a consummation of the inevitable. The marketplace currently pursues tax parity for health purchasing directly by consumers through a variety of inventive mechanisms, all of which—in attempting to work around the current tax system—add needless complexity to the entire system. The most notable and durable example is the Section 125 health plan. Under Section 125 of the tax code, employers set up "cafeteria plans" through which, according to *Health Affairs*, "Employees may purchase individual coverage with before-tax income, receiving the same tax break that exists for employer-paid premiums" (Hall, 2000). Another example is list-billing. Though specific list-billing techniques vary greatly because of state insurance law (of course), in essence they all involve a complicated administrative process through which employees select their own health plan, at individual rather than group rates, and their employers write the checks, thus preserving the tax break. Under list billing, "the insurer, rather than billing for a group rate, bills for a list of designated employees who have opted for individual coverage. This can be done in two ways," notes the *Health Affairs* analysis. "One is to bill the employer, which pays some or all of the cost of the insurance. The other is for employees to bear the entire pre-

186

mium but to allow them to pay through payroll deduction; the insurer only notifies the employer of the amounts to deduct" (Hall, 2000).

Finally, there are recurring proposals to extend to private employers like Mary's company the same cafeteria-type benefits plans available to federal employees. The Federal Employee Health Benefits Program—or "Feeb," as its acronym FEHB is pronounced—provides federal workers and their dependents in this largest of employer purchasing pools with a chunk of money for coverage. With this money, they shop for health coverage from among hundreds of competing health insurers and plans. (You know you work in a dysfunctional industry when the federal government's human resource activities are a source of innovative ideas.)

Tax parity for all Americans in purchasing their health coverage—and supplemental medical services—would create a nationwide FEHB. Under such a reform, Mary's company sets aside for her coverage exactly what it would have otherwise spent itself on funding, micromanaging, and interfering in Mary's medical care decisions. In the process, all the costs associated with her medical choices suddenly come screaming home. As we saw, Mary willingly chose a more expensive health plan that provided her and her boys freer access to the medical care they value most. This in and of itself represents a belated cultural revolution in health care consumer behavior that managed care was supposed to effect, but never did. Such a consumer cultural revolution would constitute the most powerful health care reform of all.

ERISA (OR SOMETHING LIKE IT) FOR ALL

Why will Mary's coverage be so much cheaper in 2009 than it is today? Because those three dozen insurers available to her are all free from the hodgepodge of state-based regulations that larger employers' self-funded plans are guaranteed by ERISA. The only mandated benefits that those insurers need to provide are federal ones, allowing each insurer to streamline its operations and reduce its administrative costs. This is why the national insurers Mary has access to all operate out of one headquarters location; this is also why Mary has the new option of a purely Internet-based insurer.

Determining whether this reform means literally expanding ERISA, or supplanting it with a simpler, more appropriate federal law that accomplishes the same goal, is beyond the scope of this proposal. The spirit remains the same in either case. We must do away with the arbitrary, state-by-state benefit mandates and price regulations that add increasing complexity and costs to the system and that, for all the effort, ultimately do not protect a growing segment of the insured population anyway. Such a reform will greatly reduce the organizational burdens and associated costs of running a national health insurer. And it should come with a necessary "cost" to the health insurers that in and of itself constitutes a major reform of its own: the establishment of uniform, cost of living–adjusted federal pricing regulation. Yes, Medicare pricing is too often an exercise in political extortion. But is pricing regulation at the state level any less impure? Regardless of your politics on the issue of federalism versus states' rights, by now you should recognize one overriding, if unpleasant reality: even the most onerous new federal regulations regarding mandates and premium pricing applied to everyone would be less of a burden on the system as a whole than the continued profusion of fifty-one separate, inconsistent sets of state and federal regulations.

The dissolution of state-based regulation acknowledges and accepts the market's current compulsion toward, and dexterity at, circumventing that regulation anyway. An ever-growing number of employers seek ERISA exemption for their provision of health benefits by converting to self-insurance. And the health insurers themselves have also proven adept at repackaging fully insured plans to dodge state laws. By moving toward uniform federal regulation of all health insurers, we acknowledge where the market wants to go, instead of fighting a perpetually losing battle against it. We also acknowledge the fact that a large proportion of employees with job-based insurance work for large employers with operations in more than one state. Best of all, we allow the health insurance purchasing marketplace to take full advantage of the aggressive, borderless kind of price shopping that has come to define e-commerce. When adopted in conjunction with the standardization of benefit plans described in the next section of this chapter, this long overdue legislating of marketplace realities will result in one thing: drastically lower health insurance premiums, more small employers providing coverage, and more uninsured people brought back into the system.

Despite the ambitions of the nation's state insurance commissioners, state-based regulation of health insurance is not only counterproductive but ultimately self-defeating. When a state forces more benefits down employers' throats, two things happen: a number of employers in the state go to the considerable trouble and expense of fleeing to self-insurance under ERISA, and a number of employers at the other end of the market drop coverage altogether. Mary's company is struggling with exactly this dilemma right now. More pricing and coverage mandates guarantee only that the availability of coverage shrinks. Add all these marketplace dynamics together and one thing becomes clear: the more a state tries to make specific health coverage available and affordable for its citizens, the less available and affordable it ultimately becomes.

This is especially true in the most heavily regulated of all health insurance segments, the retail market for individuals purchasing insurance with their own aftertax dollars. In an effort to stem the inevitable defections of employers subject to a state's growing number of small-group regulations—and to pick up the pieces of those defections in the retail market for individuals—health insurers have devised a variety of creative mechanisms for marketing themselves around state laws. One of the most telling is the so-called group trust. According to Mark Hall's analysis in *Health Affairs,* these legal entities "mimic the sale of large-group insurance" by creating a group to which the health insurer "issues a 'master' group policy. The insurer then sells to individuals 'certificates' under the master policy, in the same way that employees are signed up under an employer" (Hall, 2000). Group trusts circumvent state regulation as individual insurance because the policy is "issued to the trust on a group basis, and coverage is sold to individuals as certificates for members joining the group rather than as individual policies." Hall's *Health Affairs* analysis notes that "group trusts are often set up in one state to do business in several or many others. Depending on each state's treatment of jurisdictional issues, the large-group policy issued to the trust may also effectively avoid regulation as group insurance, except in the state where the trust is formed, even though certificates are sold in many other states." Confused yet? Consider what the health insurers do next in the process. According to Hall's study, they "shop among the states for the most favorable regulatory environment. This also allows insurers to create a regulatory vacuum that avoids both individual and small-group laws, since the trust is considered a large group."

Enough!

The growing number of employers taking advantage of ERISA, the success of group trust arrangements despite their obvious cumbersomeness, and ten years of consolidating health insurers into nationwide juggernauts all underscore the same point: state-based regulation of health coverage in a fluid, borderless health insurance market is antiquated, expensive, and pointless. The failure of state-by-state regulation is proven in the inverse: the widespread use of the ERISA exemption has been a success, inferred from its durability over time. We can only speculate, darkly, about how many more millions of Americans would be without insurance if ERISA were not available to employers. As Havighurst notes, "ERISA preemption has made possible a great deal of generally desirable innovation by employers and health plans that might otherwise have been precluded or discouraged by state regulation or by the threat of litigation under state law" (Havighurst, 2000, p. 92).

Because ERISA was originally intended to protect pension plans and not employers' provision of health insurance, the law is really a major loophole through all state-based laws, not a broader regulatory framework for the U.S. health system. Its usefulness, however, combined with large employer and health insurer consolidation across the country, has inspired the federal government to improve on its accidental success. The most significant of these federalist inspirations was the passage of HIPAA, which guarantees that when Mary switches from one health insurer to another, her son will not be denied coverage for his diabetes because it is a preexisting condition. Preserving portability across health insurers is particularly suitable for the "new federalism" in health care regulation; it represents the national fulfillment of what many states have tried to legislate on their own, with varying success. As Karen Pollitz observed in her analysis of HIPAA in

190

Health Affairs, the law "changed the content of consumer protections and the process of insurance regulation incrementally. One hundred twenty million Americans with private employer coverage are now less likely to have that access interrupted because of their health status, no matter where they live or their employer's size or insurance arrangement" (Pollitz, Tapay, Hadley, and Specht, 2000, p. 11).

Other equally notable laws have been passed in recent years that further overshadow state-by-state regulation of health coverage, including highly controversial mandates regarding mental health parity and minimal hospital stays for mastectomies and the delivery of babies. Emboldened by the popularity of HIPAA and these other laws, the federal government has numerous regulatory initiatives in its pipeline as of this writing, including a gusher of health insurance rules packaged for popular consumption as the "patient's bill of rights." With each new law, the federal government is establishing a set of standards that could potentially trump state-based regulation. (Unfortunately, at least in the case of HIPAA, state portability laws, where they exist, still trump the federal law.) Although one may take political issue with the content or drift of these laws, the fact that they are coming to life at the federal level, rather than among some but not all states, means that the realities of the U.S. health insurance marketplace are finally coming into focus. Their passage into federal law signals, ironically, a simpler compliance for health insurers that a crazy quilt of state laws has forever precluded.

One element that begs for such uniform regulation is price. Health insurance premium price regulation currently varies enormously by state. Some states have overt or de facto "community-rating" laws that fix prices across populations; other states have "guaranteed issue" laws that require insurers to provide coverage to all comers; still other states grind through the time-consuming and intrusive process of regulating specific premium rates for fully insured health plans, especially those marketed to individuals. This is why, as Hall notes in *Health Affairs,* "the health insurance market consists of three distinct segments, each of which is governed by fundamentally different economics and regulations: large group, small group, and individual. These are not simply points on a continuum; they constitute entirely different product lines, often sold by different sales forces and serviced by different insurers or corporate divisions—as distinct in their economic and legal characteristics as are mobile homes, condominiums, and single-family homes" (Hall, 2000). The result is the fragmentation of 50 state health insurance markets into 150 different state-level markets, all thanks to state-by-state pricing regulation.

Without such regulation, many large groups would get larger discounts than they already do, through more aggressive medical underwriting, a technique health insurers use to figure out how little they need to charge healthier groups. Small groups would get smaller or no discounts, or might pay still higher prices than they do now, penalized by medical underwriting if the group is disproportionately older, female, or blue collar. And without such regulation, individuals would take an even bigger beating. The splintering of the national health insurance market into 150 different submarkets, compelled by competitive market forces and state-based regulation, defeats the entire purpose of insurance. It encourages health insurers to pursue young, healthy workforces and price-discriminate against older ones. The result is a competitive pricing spiral that ensures that those who need insurance most are those most likely to be priced out of the market. This represents another health care market failure that ultimately benefits no one. These people swell the ranks of the uninsured and drive up costs for everybody else as they use the most costly medical services when they get sick. State-based price regulation attempts to fix this market failure in often amateurish ways, and the efforts often serve only to aggravate the problem.

If we proceed on our current course, fifty different states will continue to grapple with the dismally complex problem of pricing regulation on their own, as best they can. Those that succeed in creating new ways to level the playing field of price will succeed only in driving more employers toward ERISA or out of the provision of health insurance entirely. By contrast, if the movement toward a new federalism in health insurance continues, coupled with the universal extension of ERISA exemption or something like it to all health insurance plans, then the federal government can do the work of the fifty states in a way that would be far more sophisticated, less redundant, and less costly overall for society. My personal hope is that *all* price regulation—a ghastly, inefficient process that never really works, as in Medicare, for example—will be obviated by the other two elements of this reform proposal. The liberation of Mary's health coverage choices through tax parity and a standardization of the health insurance product will go a long way in normalizing health insurance markets, making regulation of all but the worst price discrimination unnecessary.

But such hopes may be premature. They may also prove to be naive, even if both of these other reforms are, through some miracle of political clarity, actually adopted. Although choosing a specific type of uniform price regulation is beyond the scope of this proposal, the benefits that would flow from this federalism of ultimately futile state regulations support its core argument. No matter the form it eventually takes, uniform price regulation would spare the nation's health insurers from having to cope, at great cost, with fifty state laws imposed on the national and regional marketing and administration of health insurance. It would, in effect, restore the economies of risk pooling associated with insurance that state-by-state regulation has effectively ended, as the national health insurers attempt to compete locally with smaller health insurers better positioned to cherry pick healthy populations in their own communities. It would also eliminate the onerous task of regulating and approving every little change in rates cooked up by the health insurers as they attempted to outfox each other in markets that ultimately do not work.

I am not foolish enough to believe that we can adopt this reform without political bloodshed. The doctrine of states' rights, which is legitimately applicable to matters of private property, local infrastructure, and locally transacted commerce, has numerous fans in, of all places, the federal government. (Our current president, George W. Bush, is a firm believer in the doctrine of states' rights—or at least the version of it that has been explained to him.) But that doctrine is downright useless when applied to a health care system that sprawls across borders, uses telemedicine technologies to treat patients, wants to use the Internet to conduct much of its business, and long ago adopted national clinical standards for liability. Equally strong objections to this proposed conversion to federalism for health insurance regulation will come from three places: the bureaucratic rank-and-file in

fifty state governments, the legions of health insurance company administrators that cope with those governments, and the insurance brokers that
court both to preserve their control over the health insurance distribution
channel. Again, the louder their objections, the stronger my essential argument. In presiding over—or some might say leeching off—fifty different
health care systems that apply to only two-thirds of the commercially
insured population, these three very large health care jobs programs are a
huge burden. They drain a significant portion of the 18 cents of every premium dollar that ought to be spent on good medical care for Mary, her
boys, and the uninsured in their community.

Adopting uniform federal laws to supplant the futile profusion of state
health insurance laws will be an especially bitter fight. But it is the right
fight. And I am confident that, if a belated conversion to federal regulatory
standards occurs, the best and brightest health care lobbyists currently
working in fifty statehouses will find their way to Washington. Several of
them are already *in* Washington, trying to make sense of what is going on
in all those statehouses. Without this reform, we will simply continue on
our current course, wasting a tremendous amount of money earmarked for
medical care through the passage of more and more laws that ultimately
help fewer and fewer people.

THE BENEFITS OF STANDARD BENEFITS

Flash back to the current year, and the two insurers that Mary's company
has selected for her health coverage. When their fully insured health plans
are unable to compete on price or quality, the health insurers who created
them obfuscate their unmarketability by manipulating the type and level
of medical services they will actually pay for when Mary and her boys need
them. This shell game has served the health insurers well, making it difficult if not impossible for Mary's company—not to mention Mary herself—
to price-shop for coverage. The shell game may be coming, slowly, to an
end, as evidenced by the spate of federal mandates and class-action lawsuits
against the insurers for appearing to promise one thing but actually delivering something else. But this shell game accounts for only two-thirds of

the problem. Employers who abandon the fully insured shell game using ERISA exemption, and then go on to play an even more complicated version of it with their own employees, account for the rest. Today, when a self-insured employer experiences either unforeseen cost problems or employee resistance to the ever-changing specifics of its own tailor-made benefit plan design, the employer responds with still more tailoring.

The cumulative result among both fully insured and self-insured health plans is the exponential growth of benefit plan designs across the U.S. health care system. These designs vary widely from health insurer to health insurer, from plan to plan within a health insurer's product portfolio, from self-insured employer to self-insured employer, and from plan to plan within a self-insured employers' benefits package. A chaos of inclusion rules, deductibles accounting, eligibility criteria, and coverage decisions all flow out of this colossal mess; and the most obvious question we should ask isn't why is this so difficult to administer, but rather how is anybody able to administer it at all? Mary has spent countless hours poring over the hieroglyphics of dozens of benefit-explanation letters from her current insurer, and all ultimately seem to explain only that she owes somebody more money. The eye exam for her diabetic son was covered last year; why not this year? This medication was fully covered last year; why does she have to pay for half this year?

The profusion of benefit plan designs explains why the typical health insurer spends up to 20 cents of every premium dollar designing, selling, and managing its wares. In sharp contrast, the Medicare program is able to spend 98 cents of every funded dollar on medical care. Why? Because it provides, for the most part, one standard benefit plan to 36 million beneficiaries. Although the specific features of that benefit plan are woefully out of date, the simplicity and cost efficiencies of its day-to-day claims payment processing are tremendous. Yes, much of the administrative costs of the Medicare program are off-loaded to providers as they prepare and submit claims, but exactly the same burdens exist—in a multiplicity of form—in the preparation and submission of commercial insurance claims.

The administration of one uniform benefit plan offers clear economies of scale. These economies are fully available to the major health insurers, a dozen of which have in excess of 5 million members spread across the United States. As discussed in Chapter Two, the state-based regulation of health insurance and the constant tinkering of benefit plans by employers and insurers have one overriding effect: major carriers like Aetna really consist of up to fifty little Aetnas, each with its own sprawling archipelago of benefit plan designs to manage. The process of adjudicating claims and resolving disputes across this archipelago is torturous, costly, and divisive. Nancy Dickey notes in the *New England Journal of Medicine,* "The patient-physician relationship must ultimately be one of trust, but all too often trusting relationships are disrupted not because of dissatisfaction between patient and physician but because of choices made by the patient's employer, a health insurance plan, or both" (Dickey and McMenamin, 1999, p. 1305).

This process, however disruptive and bitter, is also ultimately futile. Physicians, hospitals, patients, and their families have become, thanks to a decade of managed care, increasingly adept at working around both the specifics of health benefit designs and the eligibility rules that govern them. They recode, reclassify, and resubmit medical claims to thread through a system that by its very nature is subjective and wide open to interpretation. A large number of advocacy organizations, commercially sponsored patient assistance programs, and Internet businesses exist to help them do just this. The health insurers respond to this overrunning of their contractual authority with still more obfuscation: as providers and patients learn how to jump through each new generation of utilization management and reimbursement hoops, the insurers respond by moving the hoops around. When those hoops are placed too high, providers and patients go to court and successfully get what they were often never contractually entitled to in the first place.

This is a moronic situation. It also flies in the face of both consumer expectations and legal precedent. Regardless of what consumers and employees actually sign up for when they enroll in a specific health plan, they quickly and self-righteously attempt to supercede their agreements when they become patients months or years later. This process is reinforced by numerous legal precedents. As Havighurst notes, "It is conventional in health care law for courts to consult custom and consensus in the medical community, not specifications in private contracts, for the standards they use in defining the payment obligations of health plans in benefit disputes. Professional standards are usually viewed as binding norms, not as merely a starting point for private bargaining" (Havighurst, 2000, p. 96). The overriding authority of consumer expectations and the courts that encourage those expectations explain why health insurers—despite a thicket of language in benefits contracts—are extremely vague about how they ultimately determine benefit eligibility. "Because health plans cannot count on the courts to respect even their best efforts to authorize economizing," Havighurst writes, "today's health care contracts are largely silent about the precise content of the service packages being purchased and instead define service commitments in terms of 'medical necessity,' thereby incorporating costly professional standards by reference" (pp. 96–97).

How do we fix this problem? By reversing course, admitting the ultimately futile nature of designing ad hoc benefit plans and eligibility rules, and establishing a uniform set of health benefits consistent with the professional standards that ultimately prevail anyway. We establish, in plain view, a standard benefits plan, the one referenced in Mary's one-page policy that will go into effect in 2009. This would bring commercial health insurance administration closer to the administrative cost-ratio of the Medicare program and free up billions of health care dollars squandered on managing the current sprawl of benefit plan designs across fifty states and tens of thousands of employers.

While developing the standard benefits plan, we can and should avoid many of the problems that plague the administration of the Medicare program, which transfers numerous inefficiencies not reflected in the program's 2 cents' worth of administrative costs to providers as part of the other 98 cents paid out in claims. We do this in four ways:

- We minimize the abject politicization attendant to the process of modifying and administering the current Medicare benefits package.
- We do not dictate pricing for specific medical services under that package, leaving this to health insurers and private market forces.

- We avoid like the plague the ham-fisted enforcement of fraud and abuse laws used by Medicare to take back pennies from the 98 cents that may have been paid out in error.
- We continually refine the benefits package to avoid the near-absence of benefit design innovations that have kept much of the Medicare program in the health care equivalent of the Dark Ages.

So, how do we proceed? We create a small, nongovernmental body of health insurance experts, clinicians, actuaries, epidemiologists, and consumer advocates with one task: to design and continually modify the standard benefits plan. Despite great temptations and pressures, the plan's design should be informed entirely by science, not politics. When adopted by a critical mass of self-insured employers and health insurers, the standard benefits plan will be far less expensive to administer than any form of commercial insurance today. Why? Because of its stability, predictability, and administrative cost amortization over an enormous covered population. The resulting administrative efficiencies will attract still more employers, health insurers, and consumers, driving overall insurance costs—and thus premiums—down still further.

This kind of standardization is the health insurance equivalent of bar coding on consumer products and technical standards for fax machines. It derives its essential economies of scale by re-creating in health insurance what is known in the information technology business as Metcalfe's Law. This law dictates that the value of a standardized, networked product improves exponentially as the number of people using that type of product expands arithmetically. Such economies do not just accrue to Mary's insurance company but also represent significant cost savings for her providers. When Mary shows up at a doctor's office and presents an insurance card that says she has the standard benefits plan, the office knows exactly what is covered, what is not, and what it has to document for reimbursement.

How does this work in practice? Premiums for the standard benefits plan are funded by Mary's company or by Mary through whatever cost-sharing split they choose. Combined with the tax and regulatory reforms proposed in this chapter, the plan can be marketed directly to any consumer or employee by any health insurer in the community, or across the country. Medical services that fall outside of the plan design—be they in vitro fertilization, a Viagra prescription, or massage therapy—are purchased directly by employees. They may make such purchases out of the balance of non-taxable income "paid" to them by their employers for health care beyond the cost of premiums for the plan, they may purchase these services using tax-free income they add to this balance voluntarily (the same way flexible spending accounts work today), or they may pay out of their own pockets. This is how it will work for Mary in 2009.

Adopting the standard benefits plan will resolve many of the most bitter health insurance problems that were explored earlier in this book. In addition to the antiquated section of the tax code that favors employer-based coverage, employers are driven ever more deeply—and for the most part unhappily—into the health care business for competitive reasons. The absence of a standardized benefits plan is the reason why they are forever forced to up the ante on what they will cover if they want to retain and recruit good employees. The establishment and public promotion of the standard benefits plan across the country gives these employers a badly needed out.

"*They* decided it wasn't covered, not us," the head of Mary's human resource department can respond, each time Mary or one her coworkers asks why in vitro fertilization, or Viagra, or massage therapy is not covered. By adopting the plan, the employer is liberated, finally, from having to make moral judgments about medical services, rights, and freedoms on behalf of its employees.

Yes, adopting such a plan sounds like a move that only Big Brother could love. But the alternative, as currently practiced, is worse. Our acceptance of a standard benefits plan does away with Big Brother's seeming arbitrariness in making coverage decisions. It also means we accept the legal realities that play out in Big Brother's courts when expectations regarding health benefits go awry for sick people. Establishment of the plan will also finally put an end to the wasteful shell game played by health insurers and their brokers in the endless formulation and reformulation of plan designs.

As the plan is devised and debated by a nongovernmental entity, it will no doubt be lobbied hard from all sides of the industry; in the process it will be highly publicized by the media. When it is complete and its details are published in every major newspaper in the United States—and as it continues to be amended to incorporate medical breakthroughs—Americans will finally know, once and for all, what they are really getting for their health insurance dollars.

The creation and widespread use of the plan will reconcile much of the chronic divide between health care and medicine. It will establish a national health insurance standard that mirrors the national standards of care doctrine that has been a cornerstone of medical malpractice liability since 1975. It will also be fully consistent with how expectations about medical care are created and reinforced in American society: the national media—in its various print, broadcast, and Internet forums—will forever provide more information about what medical care works and doesn't work than any local health insurer ever has or will. One of the reasons Mary is willing to pay more for a certain insurer is its willingness to pay for any drug her son's doctors prescribe. This is important to Mary because she keeps track of new drugs for pediatric diabetes on a Web site sponsored by a national patient advocacy organization. Last year, she found out about a new one with better outcomes for children in her son's age group, a drug her son's doctor had not even heard of yet, and one her old insurer had refused to cover.

As with the supplanting of state insurance laws by federal standards, this particular reform will meet with obvious political resistance. Once again, the most ferocious objections will come from those most directly threatened by the long overdue simplification of health benefits. The enormous efficiencies flowing from widespread administration of the standard benefits plan will eat the expensive lunches of all those with vested interests in the endless tinkering of individual benefit plans. Every year, legions of benefits consultants, brokers, claims processing software companies, reimbursement vendors, and entrepreneurs of all shapes and sizes divert billions of dollars that are earmarked for medical care, as they preside over the oxymoron that is the U.S. health care "system." It's time for a *real* fix.

CHAPTER 9

Personal Effects

We'll understand it
All by and by.

From "Farther Along"
a traditional gospel folk song

When I am faced with a strong political message, my first impulse is to speculate on the prejudices and motivations of the messenger. If you are prone to the same impulse, I will save you the trouble—as some small recompense for having lasted so many pages—by providing this brief, personal coda to *Oxymorons*.

I am white, male, thirty-nine years old, well-insured, healthy, and by the standards of most Americans, financially well off. I have no formal medical training but a graduate degree in finance from Johns Hopkins, a string of publications in respected journals, and a wealth of hard experience in the health care business. Like many of my generation and professional class, I have strongly liberal views on social policy and strongly conservative views on economic policy. I am an outspoken believer in civil liberties and unfettered marketplaces, a wholly consistent political philosophy that confounds pollsters because it does not cleave to the chocolate versus vanilla of American electoral politics.

I express my political views freely at health care conferences in expensive hotels and resorts around the country. Between appearing at these conferences and running a health care software company, I travel almost constantly. I upgrade to first class, ride in taxis and limos, stay in good hotels, swap stock tips with people, hand out business cards, and spend most of my time in transit on my cell phone managing people's work and clients' expectations. I wear colorful Jerry Garcia ties, and my shirts are always pressed.

This is the image that audiences and fellow expert panel members see on the stages of those health care conferences. It prompts many on those panels—in the midst of a debate on managed care, medical economics, or patient empowerment—to challenge my views as naive and idealistic when it comes to how average Americans without insurance behave in the real world.

"You obviously do not understand poor people," the head of an academic medical center said to me during one particularly heated exchange at the Harvard School of Public Health's annual policy conference.

"That may be fine for someone with *his* income," responded a famous medical economist at another conference, "but not for the average waitress without health insurance."

"How can you say that?" the head of a health care think tank shot at me on another panel. "With your income, you don't need health insurance for any of *your* medical expenses."

I do not take issue with any of these reasonable responses to my arguments. In fact, I often catch myself thinking the same thing when I hear others championing an abstract business idea or public policy that I believe blithely dismisses real-world suffering. At the same time, I am compelled, against the caution of friends who believe doing so is foolish and risky, to explain once and forever the origins of my health care writings and the *real* health care education at the beating heart of this book. The story of health care in the United States may be an epic, but it is written one anecdote at a time. Here is mine.

Flash back to the mid-1980s, the period in our history we have come to refer to, with varying degrees of affection, as "the Reagan years." During the Reagan years—at the same age when most of my colleagues on those expert panels were earning their M.D.s and Ph.D.s—I was variously employed as a construction worker, bartender, landscaper, and cab driver. I was also, until the age of twenty-eight, a part-time college student, struggling to finish an undergraduate degree in night school. My wife at the time waited tables and worked as an office temp. She too was crawling her way toward an undergraduate degree on a part-time basis. We had no families to help us, and we tried and failed to get any real help from the government. During the Reagan years, Washington was so consumed with reducing the size of the federal government—mostly by increasing government spending to record levels, at record rates, on defense—that financial aid for tens of thousands of needy college students was one of the first things to go.

My wife and I had no health insurance. We could not afford it. In 1986, I was injured on a construction job and my wife had a series of illnesses, the combination of which consumed one-third of our $15,000 income that year. We were hounded by creditors and evicted from our tiny apartment, and moved into two rooms over a garage in a tough Baltimore neighborhood. We lived on biscuits, hot dogs, and canned corn, and washed our clothes by hand in the bathtub because we did not have money for the laundromat. We did manage, however, to scrape together a few dollars for the beer and cigarettes that dulled the constant ache of our financial struggles.

The garage in Baltimore was a damp, cold, drafty place to live, and as a result, my wife and I both developed chronic sinusitis. We could not afford to see a doctor or buy any prescriptions, but we got lucky. We medicated ourselves for nearly a year with a stash of antibiotic samples I found in the dumpster behind the medical building I cleaned for a few months for $6 per hour "cash money." Because those antibiotics had expired, their declining potency probably made our conditions worse over time by never fully clearing the infections; all we knew then was that they gave us relief from the fevers and slamming headaches. This is how poor people with no health insurance behave.

Things finally started to get better when my wife got a steady job temping for a local health insurance company. She worked there for nearly a year, typing and filing for four of the twenty-eight vice presidents of the company, each of whom she learned was making well over $100,000 per year, the equivalent of $150,000 in today's wages. According to my wife, they came in around nine o'clock every morning, wrote a memo or two for her to type and circulate, practiced putting in their offices until lunch, and spent most of the afternoon out on the golf course with local brokers, benefits consultants, and employers. Though they all liked her work, they kept her on as a temp for most of that year instead of putting her on the payroll for good reason: they did not have to provide her with costly health insurance. Premiums, you see, were going through the roof in those days.

My sister did not fare any better during the Reagan years. After struggling to finish high school, she lied about her age and started working as a cocktail waitress and eventually assistant manager of a nightclub. At age nineteen, she had no health insurance and became seriously ill. Multiple hospitalizations for a major infection resulted in bills that represented more than a third of her $20,000 gross income that year. The hospital—a Catholic-owned, not-for-profit facility with a sizable endowment and one of the highest profit margins of any hospital in the community—went after her for the bills, ruining her credit rating in the process.

My sister and I had such a difficult start in life because of our mother's own medical drama. She was born into an immigrant family that fought bitterly to establish itself in the United States against a high tide of Depression and World War II era anti-immigrant sentiment, sentiment that rises and falls but never disappears from our culture. The family's struggles were greatly complicated by my mother's diagnosis with juvenile rheumatoid arthritis (JRA) at the age of four. She spent much of her childhood in hospitals, wheelchairs, and full body casts; the only way to treat JRA in the 1940s was with aspirin, gold shots, and prolonged physical confinement. Her enormous hospital bills were all paid in full by a wealthy patron of the family, a woman my grandfather had worked for as a gardener since immigrating. This charity, according to my mother, enraged and humiliated her father, who never forgave her for her illness.

My mother eventually recovered physically. But her rage at a lost childhood was never treated. She took out this rage in the abandonment of her own children. The story of my father's life is equally painful, for different reasons but to the same end.

My sister and I survived, fighting our way out of a working poverty that persisted into our late twenties. Since then, our personal lives and professional careers have been uniquely American stories of hard work and immense grace. No help from the government, plenty of taxes then and now, and years of seventy-hour work weeks. But we owe our survival and consequent successes as much to chance (and federal charity care laws) as we do to any bogus Horatio Alger–type cultural force. Things could have gone worse. The Catholic hospital could have kicked my sister out even faster than it did; those antibiotics I found could have been exposed to the sun and killed my wife and me in one dose. And yes, we have our scars, which my sister has slowly, patiently taught me to wear with some pride, as evidenced by these words.

The many people my sister and I deal with professionally would be hard-pressed to know how hard-pressed we once were, aside from a few quirks on our resumes. My sister has a good job, good income, and lovely home, but no college degree. Of the twenty-five members of the editorial board of the policy journal, *Health Affairs*, I am one of only three without an M.D. or Ph.D. after my name. The only remaining regret from my bittersweet journey from youthful poverty to middle-aged success is purely intellectual. I did not discover any of the richness, joys, or perplexities of medicine until well into my thirties, and only as a hobby incidental to my work in health care.

I wish the story ended here: hard lessons about the U.S. health care system, learned the hard way. But the plot thickens. After a complicated pregnancy, my sister had a daughter, whom she has for the most part raised on her own. At the age of three, her daughter started to complain of pain, stiffness, and swelling in her joints—the first signs of JRA, a highly hereditary disease that tends to skip a generation. Given our mother's history, this news was an emotional earthquake for us.

Because my sister has insurance through her job, she was able to have her daughter's JRA diagnosed early and treated aggressively. And because the pharmaceutical industry has been amply rewarded for finding better ways to fight this and other hideous diseases—perhaps because the vice presidents of the nation's insurance companies are too busy playing golf with their customers to clamp down on the prices they pay for new drugs—my niece's JRA is now well-controlled with expensive Cox-2 inhibitors and one of several recent breakthrough biotech drugs. Of course, my niece's treatment has not been without the usual struggles. My sister's health insurer made every effort to block her daughter's access to the best pediatric rheumatologist in their community, defined for my layperson sister and this health information professional alike as the specialist recommended most enthusiastically by every primary care doctor in our town. Her insurer also made every effort to block her access to the best drugs for treating her condition, especially the Cox-2 inhibitor, even after my sister and the rheumatologist provided extensive documentation that the older pain medications the insurer insisted on were upsetting my eight-year-old niece's stomach to the point where she was vomiting several times every day. (This same insurer's TV ads that year ended with "quality health care for your whole family.")

Despite my niece's JRA and her health insurer's best efforts, she is healthy, happy, and athletic. She has recovered to the point where she can compete in gymnastics and swimming. She plays music, skis, bikes, hikes, and loves to run across the room and slam-tackle her uncle when she sees him walk through the door. I cannot confirm if my niece's doctors are any better than my mother's were. What I can confirm is this: the only verifiable difference between the joyfulness of my niece's childhood and the living nightmare that was my mother's—aside from the fickleness of any disease's progression—are five decades of costly pharmaceutical research.

That is the wellspring of my health care politics. From these painful personal experiences, I have my own evidence for one unassailable conclusion. The only progress we make in health care is the progress we make in medicine. In the daily chaos that is the U.S. health care "system," there are but three elements that matter: patients, caregivers, and medical technologies. Everything else is noise.

REFERENCES

Anderson, G., Greenberg, G., and Lisk, C. K. "Academic Health Centers: Exploring a Financial Paradox." *Health Affairs,* 1999, *18*(2), 156–164.

Armstrong, L., and Jenkins, S. *It's Not About the Bike.* New York: Putnam, 2000.

Arnold, W. "Letter to the Editor." *Modern Healthcare,* Oct. 16, 2000, p. 72.

Ayanian, J., and others. "Unmet Health Needs of Uninsured Adults in the United States." *JAMA,* 2000, *284,* 2061–2069.

Baker, P., and others. "Impact of Patient-with-Patient Interaction on Perceived Rheumatoid Arthritis Overall Disease Status." *Scandinavian Journal of Rheumatology,* 1996, *25*(4), 207–212.

Becker, C. "The Scope of the Debate." *Modern Healthcare,* Aug. 7, 2000, p. 52. [www.modernhealthcare.com]

Bell, C. "Follow the Money." *Modern Healthcare,* Oct. 23, 2000, p. 22.

Bellandi, D. "Florida Hospital, Alliance Part Ways." *Modern Healthcare,* Oct. 30, 2000a, pp. 24–25.

Bellandi, D. "Hospital Prices Jump." *Modern Healthcare,* Nov. 13, 2000b, p. 4.

Bellandi, D. "Reports Paint Differing Conversion Portraits." *Modern Healthcare,* Nov. 13, 2000c, pp. 8–10.

Benko, L. "Few Follow United's Lead." *Modern Healthcare,* Aug. 14, 2000, p. 2.

Bennehum, D. "The Hot New Medium Is. . .E-Mail." *Wired.* Apr. 1998, p. 104–106.

Bentivoglio, J. "Unleash the Internet." *Modern Healthcare,* Nov. 6, 2000, p. 76.

Billings, J., Parikh, N., and Mijanovich, T. "Emergency Department Use in New York City: A Substitute for Primary Care?" *The Commonwealth Fund,* Nov. 2000a, pp. 1–5.

Billings, J., Parikh, N., and Mijanovich, T. "Emergency Room Use: The New York Story." *The Commonwealth Fund,* Nov. 2000b, pp. 1–11.

Blue Cross and Blue Shield Association of America. "State Mandated Benefits and Providers. Part I." Chicago: Blue Cross and Blue Shield Association of America, 2000.

Blumenstein, R. "Auto Makers Attack High Health-Care Bills with a New Approach." *Wall Street Journal,* Dec. 9, 1996, p. A1.

Bodenheimer, T. "Executives with White Coats—The Work and World View of Managed-Care Medical Directors. Part I." *New England Journal of Medicine*, Dec. 16, 1999, *341*(25), 1945–1948.

Bodenheimer, T., and Casalino, L. "Executives with White Coats—The Work and World View of Managed-Care Medical Directors. Part II." *New England Journal of Medicine*, Dec. 23, 1999, *341*(26). [www.nejm.org]

Brannigan, M. "Congress's Removal of 'Slots' Opened a Flood at New York Airport's Gates." *Wall Street Journal, Interactive Edition*, Dec. 4, 2000. [www.wsj.com]

Buck, J., Teich, J. L., Umland, B., and Stein, M. "Behavioral Health Benefits in Employer-Sponsored Health Plans." 1997, *Health Affairs*, 1999, *18*(2), 67–90.

Burton, T. "Self-Examination: An HMO Checks Up on Its Doctors' Care and Is Disturbed Itself." *Wall Street Journal*, July 8, 1998, p. A1.

"California Health Insurer's Online Marketing Plan Angers Brokers." *IMMS Daily Newsletter*, Feb. 14, 2000. [www.imms.com]

Carrns, A. "GM Enters Pact to Promote Use of Medscape's Electronic Systems." *Wall Street Journal*, Jan. 26, 2001. [www.wsj.com]

Christensen, C., Bohmer, R., and Kenagy, J. "Will Disruptive Innovations Cure Health Care?" *Harvard Business Review*, Sept.–Oct. 2000, p. 103–111.

Comparative Performances of U.S. Hospitals: The Sourcebook. 1992–1998 editions. Baltimore, Md.: HCIA, all years.

Cooper, B., and Vladeck, B. C. "Bringing Competitive Pricing to Medicare." *Health Affairs*, 2000, *19*(5), 49–56.

Cutillo, B. "Teaching Professionalism to Medical Students" (Letter to the Editor). *JAMA*, 2000, *283*(2), 197.

Dallek, G., and Swersky, L. "Comparing Medicare HMOs: Do They Keep Their Members?" *Families USA Foundation*, Dec. 1997. [www.familiesusa.org]

Deming, W. E. *Out of the Crisis.* Cambridge, Mass.: Center for Advanced Engineering Study, Massachusetts Institute of Technology, 1982.

Devine, E. "Meta-Analysis of the Effects of Psychoeducational Care in Adults with Asthma." *Residential Nursing Health*, 1996, *19*(5), 367–376.

Dickey, N., and McMenamin, P. "Putting Power into Patient Choice." *New England Journal of Medicine*, 1999, *31*(17), 1305–1307.

"Doctors Test Electronic Implant Designed to Fight Depression." *Wall Street Journal Interactive Edition*, Nov. 27, 2000. [www.wsj.com]

Dubois, R., and others. "Explaining Drug Spending Trends." *Health Affairs*, 1998, *19*(2), 231–239.

Dudley, R., Miller, R. H., Korenbrot, T. Y., and Luft, H. S. "The Impact of Financial Incentives on Quality of Health Care." *Milbank Quarterly*, 1998, *76*(4), 649–686.

Erickson, L., and others. "The Relationship Between Managed Care Insurance and Use of Lower Mortality Hospitals for CABG Surgery." *JAMA*, 2000, *283*(15). [online edition, Apr. 19, 2000]

"Federal Agency States Decision on Birth Control, Health Coverage." *Wall Street Journal,* Dec. 14, 2000. [www.wsj.com]

Fein, F. "Doctors Maintain Connection with Patients Through E-Mail." *The New York Times,* Nov. 20, 1997. [www.nytimes.com]

"Finding Medical Help Online." *Consumer Reports,* Feb. 1997, pp. 27–31.

"Former Charter CEO Heads Iasis Division." *Modern Healthcare,* Nov. 20, 2000, p. 20.

Freudenheim, M. "Six Health Plans Are Developing Online Venture." *The New York Times,* Mar. 30, 2000. [www.nytimes.com]

Fronstin, P., and Helman, R. "Small Employers and Health Benefits: Findings from the 2000 Small Employer Health Benefits Survey." *EBRI Issue Brief No. 226 and Special Report SR 35,* Oct. 2000, 1–20.

Fuchs, V. "Health Care for the Elderly: How Much? Who Will Pay for It?" *Health Affairs,* Jan.-Feb. 1999, *18*(1), 11.

Gabel, J., Hunt, K. A., and Hurst, K. "When Employers Choose Health Plans: Do NCQA Accreditation and HEDIS Data Count?" *Commonwealth Fund,* Sept. 1998. [www.cmwf.org]

"Gain-Sharing Illegal." *Modern Healthcare,* July 12, 1999. [www.modernhealthcare.com]

Galewitz, P. "Online Health Spending to Soar." *Associated Press,* Jan. 26, 2000. [http://news.excite.com/news/ap/000126/00/online-health]

Glasser, R. "The Doctor Is Not In." *Harper's,* Mar. 1998, pp. 35–41.

Gleick, J. *Chaos.* New York: Penguin Books, 1987.

Goldberger, A. "Non-Linear Dynamics for Clinicians: Chaos Theory, Fractals, and Complexity at the Bedside." *The Lancet,* 1996, *347,* 1312–1314.

Goldberger, A., Bhargava, V., West, B. J., and Mandell, A. "On a Mechanism of Cardiac Electrical Stability: The Fractal Hypothesis." *Biophysics Journal,* 1985, *48,* 525.

Goldsmith, J. "How Will the Internet Change Our Health System?" *Health Affairs,* 2000, *19*(1). [www.healthaffairs.org]

"The Great Consolidator." *Modern Healthcare,* Feb. 21, 2000. [www.modern-healthcare.com]

Grimes, T. Letter to the Editor. *Modern Healthcare,* Oct. 16, 2000, p. 72.

Hall, M. "The Geography of Health Insurance Regulation: A Guide to Identifying, Exploiting, and Policing Market Boundaries." *Health Affairs,* 2000, *19*(2), 173–182. [www.healthaffairs.org]

Havighurst, C. "American Health Care and the Law—We Need to Talk!" *Health Affairs,* 2000, *19*(4), 84–106.

HCIA Guide to the Managed Care Industry. 1995–1998 editions. Baltimore, Md.: HCIA, all years.

HCIA National Inpatient Profile. 1992–1998 editions. Baltimore, Md.: HCIA, all years.

Health Data Directory. New York: Faulkner & Gray, 2000.

"HMOs." *Modern Healthcare,* Feb. 15, 1999, p. 52.

Jaklevic, M. "Wanted: A Few Good Leaders." *Modern Healthcare,* Oct. 2, 2000a, pp. 38–40.

Jaklevic, M. "Trouble on the Margins." *Modern Healthcare,* Dec. 4, 2000b, p. 2.

Jesitus, J. "Conceiving Infertility Benefits." *Managed Healthcare,* Nov. 2000, p. 16.

Johnson, S. "Strategic Planning? Try Strategic Doing." *Modern Healthcare,* Aug. 14 2000, p. 48.

Kaiser Family Foundation. "Americans as Healthcare Consumers: The Role of Quality Information." Menlo Park, Calif.: Henry J. Kaiser Family Foundation, 1996.

Kaiser Family Foundation (and Health Research and Educational Trust). "Employer Health Benefits 2000 Annual Survey." Menlo Park, Calif.: Henry J. Kaiser Family Foundation, 2000.

Kazemek, E. "Wanted: Courageous Leadership." *Modern Healthcare,* Aug. 21, 2000, p. 36.

King, R. "FTC Widens Probe into Generic Drug Barriers." *Wall Street Journal,* Mar. 9, 1999a, p. B1.

King, R. "McKesson Restates 4th Period Results." *Wall Street Journal,* Apr. 29, 1999b, p. A3.

Kirchheimer, B. "Alike Yet Different." *Modern Healthcare,* Jul. 5, 1999, pp. 26–27.

Kirchheimer, B. "Nashville Healthcare's Patron." *Modern Healthcare,* Nov. 6, 2000a, pp. 52–53.

Kirchheimer, B. "The Street Takes a Positive Second Look." *Modern Healthcare,* Nov. 6, 2000b, p. 81.

Kleinke, J. *Bleeding Edge: The Business of Health Care in the New Century.* Gaithersburg, Md.: Aspen, 1998a.

Kleinke, J. "Paradigm Lost: Deconstructing the Columbia/HCA Investigation." *Health Affairs,* 1998b, *17*(2), 7–26.

Kleinke, J. "Release 0.0: Information Technology in the Real World." *Health Affairs,* 1998c, *17*(6), 23.

Kohn, L. T., Corrigan, J. M., and Donaldson, M. S. (eds.). *To Err Is Human: Building a Safer Health System.* Washington, D.C.: Committee on Quality of Health Care in America, Institute of Medicine, National Academy Press, 2000.

Kronick, R., and Gilmer, T. "Explaining the Decline in Health Insurance Coverage, 1979–1995." *Health Affairs,* 1999, *18*(2), 30–47.

Kuttner, R. "Must Good HMOs Go Bad? Part I: The Search for Checks and Balances." *New England Journal of Medicine,* 1998a, *338*(21), 1559–1563.

Kuttner, R. "Must Good HMOs Go Bad? Part II: The Search for Checks and Balances." *New England Journal of Medicine,* 1998b, *338*(22). [www.nejm.org]

Laster, L. "It's Not the Job." *Washington Post,* Feb. 21, 2001. [online edition]

Lee-Feldstein, A., Feldstein, P. J., Buchmueller, T., and Katterhagen, G. "The Relationship of HMOs, Health Insurance, and Delivery Systems to Breast Cancer Outcomes." *Medical Care,* 2000, *38,* 705–718.

Lewis, M. *The New New Thing*. New York: Norton, 2000.

Lieberman, D., and others. "Use of Colonoscopy to Screen Asymptomatic Adults for Colorectal Cancer." *New England Journal of Medicine*, 2000, *343*(3). [www.nejm.org]

Lieu, T. A., and others. "Projected Cost-Effectiveness of Pneumococcal Conjugate Vaccination of Healthy Infants and Young Children." *JAMA*, 2000, *283*(11), 1460–1468.

Lovern, E. "New Sharps Law May Stick Some Providers." *Modern Healthcare*, Nov. 14, 2000a, p. 6.

Lovern, E. "The Right Ratio." *Modern Healthcare*, Oct. 16, 2000b, pp. 3, 10.

Lovern, E. "Some Catch a Break on Oryx Requirements." *Modern Healthcare*, Nov. 6, 2000c, pp. 2–3.

Lovern, E. "The PPO Accreditation Contest." *Managed Healthcare*, Jan. 29, 2001, pp. 4–5.

Marshall, J. "Complexity, Chaos, and Incomprehensibility: Parsing the Biology of Critical Illness." *Critical Care Medicine*, 2000, *28*(7), 2646–2648.

Martinez, B. "Business Consortium to Launch Effort Seeking Higher Standards at Hospitals." *Wall Street Journal Interactive Edition*, Nov. 15, 2000. [www.wsj.com]

McClellan, M., McNeil, B. J., and Newhouse, J. P. "Does More Intensive Treatment of Acute Myocardial Infarction in the Elderly Reduce Mortality? Analysis Using Variables." *JAMA*, 1994, *272*(11), 859–866.

McCormick, D., and others. "Differences in Discharge Medication After Acute Myocardial Infarction in Patients with HMO and Fee-for-Service Medical Insurance." *Journal of General Internal Medicine*, 1999, *14*(2), 73–81.

McCue, M. "Consumer Governed, Patient Focused." *Managed Healthcare Executive*, Oct. 21, 1998, p. 14.

McDonald, C. "Canopy Computing: Using the Web in Clinical Practice." *JAMA*, 1998, *280*(15), 1325–1329.

Mechanic, D. "Managed Care and the Imperative for a New Professional Ethic." *Health Affairs*, 2000, *19*(5), 102–103.

Miller, T., and Reents, S. "The Health Care Industry in Transition: The Online Mandate to Change." Cyber Dialogue (on behalf of Intel), July 1998. [www.cyberdialogue.com/pdfs/wp/wp-cch-1999-transition.pdf]

Morrissey, J. "Internet Dominates Providers' Line of Sight." *Modern Healthcare*, Apr. 10, 2000, pp. 72–86.

Mort, E. A., and others. "Physician Response to Patient Insurance Status in Ambulatory Care Clinical Decision-Making: Implications for Quality of Care." *Medical Care*, 1996, *8*, 783–797.

Mullan, F. "The Case for More U.S. Medical Students." *New England Journal of Medicine*, 2000, *343*(3), 213–217.

Navarro, R. "Managed Care Forum: Forecasting Issues for Managed Care Pharmacy." *American Journal of Health Systems Pharmacists*, Jan. 1, 1998, *55*, 27.

Nguyen, N. X., and Derrick, F. W. "Hospital Markets and Competition: Implications for Antitrust Policy." In M. Brown (ed.), *Integrated Health Care Delivery: Theory, Practice, Evaluation, and Prognosis.* Gaithersburg, Md.: Aspen, 1996, p. 213.

Nuland, S. "The Hazards of Hospitalization." *Wall Street Journal,* Dec. 2, 1999.

"Outliers." *Modern Healthcare,* Jan. 1, 2001, p. 40.

"Painful Pursuit of a Competitive Marketplace." *Health Affairs,* 2000, *19*(5), 6, 84–102.

Passi, G. "Chaos Theory and Medicine." *National Medical Journal of India,* 1999, *12*(3), 93–95.

Pauly, M., and others. "Measuring Community Benefits Provided by For-Profit and Nonprofit Hospitals." *Health Affairs,* 2000, *19*(6), 168–177.

Peeno, L. "What Is the Value of a Voice?" *U.S. News,* Mar. 9, 1998. [www.usnews.com]

Phillips, K. A., Mayer, M. L., and Aday, L. "Barriers to Care Among Racial/Ethnic Groups Under Managed Care." *Health Affairs,* 2000, *19*(4), 65–75.

"PHOs Losing Steam." *Modern Healthcare,* June 6, 1998. [www.modernhealthcare.com]

Pollitz, K., Tapay, N., Hadley, E., and Specht, J. "Early Experience with 'New Federalism' in Health Insurance Regulation." *Health Affairs,* 2000, *19*(4), 8–20.

Rauber, C. "HMO Study Finds $768 Million Loss." *Modern Healthcare,* Sept. 7, 1998, 24, 30.

Ray, W., Gigante, J., Mitchel, E. F., and Hickson, G. B. "Perinatal Outcomes Following Implementation of TennCare." *JAMA,* 1998, *279*(4), 314–316.

Reinhardt, U. "The Economics of For-Profit and Nonprofit Hospitals." *Health Affairs,* 2000, *19*(6), 178.

Reschovsky, J. D., Kemper, P., and Tu, H. "Does Type of Health Insurance Affect Health Care Use and Assessments of Care Among the Privately Insured?" *Health Services Research,* 2000, *35*, 219–237.

Robertson, K. "Are Health Plan Brokers Paid Too Much?" *Sacramento Business Journal,* Sept. 13, 1999. [http://bizjournals.bcentral.com/sacramento/stories/1999/09/13story4.html]

Roetzheim, R., and others. "Effects of Health Insurance and Race on Colorectal Cancer Treatments and Outcomes." *American Journal of Public Health,* 2000, *90*(11), 1746–1754.

Rundle, R. "Calpers Rejects 2002 Health-Care Bids as Too High and Asks for Resubmission." *Wall Street Journal,* Feb. 23, 2001. [www.wsj.com]

Russell, L. *Is Prevention Better Than the Cure?* Washington, D.C.: Brookings Institution, 1986.

Safran, D. G., Tarlov, A. R., and Rogers, W. H. "Primary Care Performance in Fee-for-Service and Prepaid Health Care Systems. Results from the Medical Outcomes Study." *JAMA,* 1994, *271*(20), 1579–1586.

Safran, D. G, and others. "Organizational and Financial Characteristics of Health Plans: Are They Related to Primary Care Performance?" *Archives of Internal Medicine*, 2000, *160*(1), 69–76.

Schoen, C., and DesRoches, C. "Uninsured and Unstably Insured: The Importance of Continuous Insurance Coverage." *Health Services Research*, Apr. 2000, *35*, 187–206.

Schultz, E., and others. "Firms Are Using Trust Funds to Pay Retiree Benefits, Boosting Bottom Line." *Wall Street Journal Interactive Edition*, Oct. 25, 2000. [www.wsj.com]

"Second-Class Medicine." *Consumer Reports*, Sept. 2000. [www.consumerreports.com]

Sells, S. "Squeezing the Middleman." *Healthcare Business*, May 2000. [www.healthcarebusiness.com]

Sheils, J., and Hogan, P. "Cost of Tax-Exempt Health Benefits in 1998." *Health Affairs*, 1999, *18*(2), 177–179.

Sherman, V. "Wrong People for the Job?" *Modern Healthcare*, Nov. 20, 2000, p. 28.

Silicon Alley Reporter, as reported by the Associated Press, April 27, 2000.

Soumerai, S., and others. "Timeliness and Quality of Care for Elderly Patients with Acute Myocardial Infarction Under Health Maintenance Organization vs. Fee-for-Service Insurance." *Archives of Internal Medicine*, 1999, *159*, 2013–2020.

Starr, P. *The Social Transformation of American Medicine*. NY: Basic Books, 1982.

Starr, P. "Smart Technology, Stunted Policy: Developing Health Information Networks." *Health Affairs*, 1997, *15*(3), 91–105.

Stingl, J. "Giving Thanks for Life Itself." *JSOnline* (*Milwaukee Journal Sentinel*), Nov. 21, 2000. [www.jsonline.com]

Sullivan, K. "On the 'Efficiency' of Managed Care Plans." *Health Affairs*, 2000, *19*(4), 139–148.

Tamblyn, R., and others. "Association Between Licensing Examination Scores and Resource Use and Quality of Care in Primary Care Practice." *JAMA*, 1998, *280*(11), 989–995.

Taylor, M. "Unusual Deal Saves Alabama Hospital." *Modern Healthcare*, Oct. 18, 1999, p. 26.

Taylor, M. "Medicare Overpaid Health Plans." *Modern Healthcare*, Sept. 25, 2000, p. 6.

Taylor, M. "HCA Settlement Looms Large." *Modern Healthcare*, Jan. 1, 2001, p. 31.

Waldholz, M., and Moore, S. "Glaxo SmithKline Plans to Market Drugs Over the Internet and Exploit R&D Heft." *Wall Street Journal*, Jan. 18, 2000, p. A3.

Walker, T. "Length-of-Stay Care Guidelines Face Scrutiny." *Managed Healthcare*, Nov. 2000, pp. 10–11.

Ware, J. Jr. "Differences in 4-Year Health Outcomes for Elderly and Poor, Chronically Ill Patients Treated in HMO and Fee-for-Service Systems." *JAMA*, 1996, *276*(1), 1039–1047.

Wechsler, J. "Senate Sneaks in Modest Patients' Rights Legislation." *Managed Health-care*, Aug. 2000, p. 15.

Winslow, R., and Hensley, S. "New Treatment for Heart Disease Nears Approval." *Wall Street Journal*, Nov. 3, 2000, pp. B1, B4.

Winslow, R., and Hensley, S. "High Tech Cardiac Care Finds Support in Study." *Wall Street Journal Interactive Edition*, Nov. 16, 2000.

INDEX

Clinical experience, reliance on, 119
Clinical gain, 76
Clinical guidelines, 61–62, 64, 118, 124
Clinical information, 151–154, 155
Clinical outcomes, 68, 105, 110, 120, 121; comparing, 60, 61
Clinical practice control systems, imposition of, 118–119
Clinical standards, national, adoption of, 193
Clinical variation, 20–21
Clinton administration, 16, 114
Clinton Health Care Reform Plan, 17, 66, 79, 183
Closed clinical IT systems, 151
Cognitive compromises, 118–119, 125
Collection efforts, effect of, 169
Collective health status, investment in, 25
Collective unconscious preference, 169–170
Colon cancer, 61, 77
Colonoscopies, 77, 78
Columbia, 98, 99
Columbia-HCA, persecution of, 18
Commercial health insurance, 2, 3
Commercial managed care, notion of, 72
Commission on Medicaid and the Uninsured, 173
Commissions, 48, 182
Commonwealth Fund, 168
Community health clinics, 166, 174–175
Community Health Information Networks (CHINS), 134, 135, 145
Community Health Systems, 98, 99
Community hospitals, 101; construction of, 85–90; management of, 92–98; scenario involving, 83–84
Community rating, 70, 191
Comparative Performances of U.S. Hospitals: The Sourcebook, 87
Compensation models, 11
Competition, 20, 86, 171–172
Competitive bidding, 17, 71
Competitive pricing, resistance to, 89
Complexity theory, 109, 119, 120, 121–124, 128–130, 148; applicability

of, 110, 112–113; core tenet of, 111; and data results, 125–126, 127; development of, 111–112; examples illustrating, 113–115, 117–118; principles of, 112, 113–117
Compliance, 21–22
Compulsory charity, notion of, 170
Connectivity, 134, 135, 136, 137, 140–146, 148. *See also* Internet connectivity
Connectivity companies, 104, 105, 134–135, 136, 148, 151, 158. *See also* Internet connectivity companies
Conservative companies, 30
Consolidated Omnibus Budget Reconciliation Act (COBRA), 39
Consolidation, 9, 12, 16, 42–43, 190
Consultants, 94, 97, 104, 105, 183
Consulting companies, 97–98, 104, 105
Consulting processes, 128
Consumer advocates, 40–41
Consumer behavior. *See* Consumer culture
Consumer choice, 71, 139, 156, 179, 185, 193. *See also* Health care reform
Consumer coalitions, hampering of, 8
Consumer culture, 2, 79, 80, 122, 123, 159, 187
Consumer demand, 7, 21, 28, 151; causes of, 4, 152, 155, 159; responsibility for, 74–75, 77–78, 153
Consumer empowerment, 153, 200
Consumer expectations, 13, 20, 45–46, 196–197, 199
Consumer health care information, 4, 46, 77, 151–159
Consumer medical choices, 40, 122, 159, 187
Consumer mobility, 40, 185
Consumer Reports, 152, 157, 169, 173, 175
Consumerism and the Goldfarb ruling, 13
Consumers: becoming patients, 77; nature of, 2. *See also under specific topics*
Continuing education, 96
Continuity of care, 63, 169, 179
Continuous coverage, 39–42, 179–180
Contraceptives, 44, 47

Drugs, newer and better, 36, 58, 73, 76
Drugstore.com, 137
Dubois, R., 155
Dudley, R., 60
Duke University, 5

E

Early diagnosis, 61
E-commerce, advantage of, 188
E-communities, 154
Economic alignment, 11–12, 103, 147
Economic conflicts, 51, 135, 146, 147, 160;
    between employer and employee, 40,
    41, 91
Economic disconnection, 10, 72, 140
Economic interests, threat to, 183
Economies of scale, 74, 195–196, 198
EDS, 54
Electronic claims processing, 45, 141–142,
    145
Electronic Medical Records (EMRs), 134,
    135, 148
Eligibility criteria, 195, 197
E-mail communication, 160
E-mail visits, 159–161
Emergency Medical Treatment and Active
    Labor Act (EMTALA), 170
Emergency room service, 44, 167, 168,
    169, 170; scenarios involving, 148–150,
    165–166
Emergency rooms, status of, 174–175
Emergent conditions, treating, 166, 168
Employee Benefits Research Institute
    (EBRI), 180
Employee flexible spending accounts, 185
Employee medical records, abuse of,
    37–38
Employee Retirement Income Security Act
    (ERISA), 5–6, 13, 29, 37, 42; divide cre-
    ated by, 43; expanding or supplanting,
    187–188, 192; seeking exemption
    through, 44, 188, 189, 190, 195
Employer purchasers, 32, 51, 52, 88, 140
Employer-based coverage: amount spent
    on, 28; decline in, 29; fundamental
    problem of, 30; idea of, scenario on, 1

Employer-based payment system, begin-
    nings of, 2, 3–4, 28
Employer-based retirement funding, 185
Employer-employee economic conflict,
    40, 41, 91
Employers: expectations of, 69; hampering
    of, 8; imposition of, 2, 3, 51, 91–92; lib-
    eration of, 199. *See also under specific
    topics*
Employers, self-insured. *See* Self-insured
    employers
Employment data, 38–39
End stage renal disease (ESRD) contract-
    ing, scenario involving, 83–84
End-of-life care, 30, 31, 36
Enrollment, 69–70, 71, 180
Enterprisewide systems, 134
Enthoven, A., 65
Entitlement. *See* Medical care entitlement
Envoy, 135, 145
Equal Employment Opportunity Com-
    mission, 47
Equifax, 144
Equilibrium, 22, 113, 115–116
Equilibrium pricing point, 40
Erickson, L., 157
Escrowed premiums, 182
Eskind family, 98
Ethical responsibilities, conflict with, 2
Evidence-based medicine, 68
E-visits, reimbursement for, 160
Express Scripts, 136

F

Fairfield Health Industry Authority, 87
"Federal Agency States Decision on Birth
    Control, Health Coverage," 44, 47
Federal budget, 19
Federal court rulings, 48. *See also* U.S.
    Supreme Court
Federal Employee Health Benefits (FEHB)
    Program, 187
Federal Express, 54, 55
Federal regulation. *See specific regulations
    and mandates*
Federal Reserve Board, 129

Havighurst, C., 5, 22, 30, 45, 88, 170, 184, 190, 196–197
HBO & Company (HBOC), 134–135, 137, 148, 162, 163
HCA, The Healthcare Company, 18, 98, 99
HCIA, 38, 124, 126, 137, 147, 157, 158, 162
HCIA Guide to the Managed Care Industry, 71
HCIA National Inpatient Profile, 76
Health Affairs, 17, 20, 29, 47, 89, 90, 99, 102, 104, 126, 156, 184, 186, 189, 191, 205
Health benefit mandates, 29, 42–47, 48, 50, 91, 188, 189; beginning of, 5, 6
Health benefit plan designs, 29, 40, 91, 195; proliferation of, 142, 181, 182, 195. *See also* Standard benefits plan
Health benefits: decisions on, measuring impact of, 36–37, 38–39; disputes over, 196–197; management of, 29–30, 31–32, 34; vicious cycle of, 91–92
Health care: inability to rationalize, 128; versus medicine, 104; physician training in, 105, 106; progress in, defining, 206; underlying fact of, 108–109
Health care administration programs, lack of, 96
Health care costs, total. *See* U.S. health care expenditures
Health Care Financing Administration (HCFA), 75, 127, 130, 142, 158, 160
Health care industry: lack of self-knowledge in, 125–126; paradox of, 85–86
Health care information companies, pre-Internet. *See* Connectivity companies
Health care jobs program. *See* Middle-class jobs program
Health care management departments, creation of, 35–36
Health care reform, 17, 24, 85; objections to, source of, 183, 200; principle goals of, reasons for, 178–180; and simplification, 181–182; through a standard benefits plan, 181, 194–200; through federalism, 181, 187–194; through tax parity, 25, 182, 184–187

Health care rhetoric gap, 156, 157
Health care vendors, interests of, 183
Health Insurance Association of America, 157
Health insurance brokers, 2, 48–50, 49, 182, 183, 193
Health insurance coverage: continuous, 39–42, 179–180; disruption in, 39–40, 179; loss of, 25, 37, 179, 189; purchasing, 29–30, 49, 50, 187
Health insurance market segments, fragmentation of, 191–192
Health insurance portability, 6, 47, 181; mandating, 38, 39, 41, 190, 191
Health Insurance Portability and Accountability Act (HIPAA), 38, 39, 41, 47, 141, 190–191
Health insurance premiums, 71, 90, 182, 188; for self-insured employers, 43–44; unaffordable, 166, 167, 180. *See also* *Price entries*
Health insurer administrators, resistance from, 193
Health insurers: battling with, 94, 206; choice of, 39; consolidation of, 12, 190; imposition of, 2; profits of, 182; secret of, 145; selection of, 39, 40; virtualized, 156. *See also* *under specific topics*
Health maintenance organizations (HMOs), 34–35, 55, 58; comparing, to fee-for-service, 60, 61, 62–63
Health Management Associates, 98
Health marts, 159
Health Network, The, 157
Health plans: consolidation of, 42–43; difference among, scenario involving, 27–28; performance of, 157; policies of, 48–49; selection of, 34–35, 156–157, 177–178, 185, 186. *See also specific types*
Health Services Research, 62, 64, 179
Health status, 25, 60, 68
Healtheon, 135, 139, 140–141, 143, 145, 146
HealthGrades.com, 157
HealthMont, 99
Healthplan Employer Data and Information Set (HEDIS), 35, 157

HealthTrust, 98, 99
Heart attack, 61–62, 75, 79, 80, 121
Heart disease, 68, 73, 75; scenario involving, 107–108
Heart surgery, 75, 76
Heart-rate variability, 116–117
Helman, R., 14, 41, 180
Hensley, S., 75
Hickson, G. B., 60
Hierarchy of needs, 74
High-quality and low-cost issues. See Cost-quality conundrum
High-risk pregnancy detection and management, 36
Hill, T., 99
Hill-Burton program, 86–87
Hiring practices, 38
Hispanics, 61
HIV/AIDS, 31, 37, 120, 126
HMO Act, 56
"HMOs," 11
Hogan, P., 28, 184
Home Depot, 54
Homeostasis, return to, 120
Hospice care, 30, 44, 122
Hospital administrators, 92–94, 96, 100, 101, 105, 106
Hospital capacity, 85, 86–87, 89
Hospital chains, 95, 98–101
Hospital decision making, involving physicians in, 84, 101, 103; scenario involving, 83–84
Hospital industry: fragmentation in, 95; and profitability, 19, 104
Hospital management, 9–10, 93–96, 100–101, 103
Hospital ownership, 9, 98, 100, 126
Hospital trust fund, 127
Hospital-physician alignment, 11–12, 103
Hospital-physician integration, 7, 12, 146–151
Hospital-physician relationship, 10, 11–12, 101, 102, 103, 104
Hospitals: closure of, 87; competition among, 86; construction of, 87–88; control over, beginning of, 55; integra-

tion between, 7–8; larger, assumption made by, 102; paradox of, 94; purchasing by, 100, 103; types of, 95. See also under specific topics and types
Human anatomy and physiology, complexity of, 116–118
Human genome project, 74
Human resource departments, 29–30, 31, 41
Hunt, K. A., 35, 157
Huntington's disease, 154
Hurst, K., 35, 157
Hybrid system, 13, 20, 74

I

Iasis, 99–100
Imaging, breakthroughs in, 73
Immunization, 67–68, 81
In vitro fertilization, 29, 30, 31, 37, 47, 198–199; scenario involving, 27–28
Inclusion rules, 195
Indemnity insurance, 55, 63. See also Fee-for-service
Independent practice associations (IPAs), 8, 147
Individual policies, 191
Inertia Factor, 8, 48, 50, 74; presence of, 16, 21, 70, 91
Infertility treatments, 44
Inflation, 28–29, 155
Information databases, origins of, 140
Information software and complexity theory, 128
Information system integration. See Connectivity
Information systems, benefits of, 134
Information systems (IT) vendors. See Connectivity companies; Internet connectivity companies
Information technology (IT): adopting, barriers to, 45, 148, 151; costs of, 33; reliability of, 150–151; spending on, 137–138. See also Connectivity; Internet connectivity
Inpatient care, cost of, 94
Inpatient supply and demand, 85

O

OASIS regulations, 130
Off-budget public expenditure, 184
Office visits, 159–161
OnHealth, 135
On-line pharmacies, 136
On-line support groups, 154
Open access to legacy databases, 144
Open computing technology, 148, 151. *See also* Internet-based computing; Internet connectivity
Open-access plans, devolving to, 40
OrNda, 98
Outcome measurement and complexity theory, 120, 121
Outcomes and inputs, 110, 112, 128. *See also* Complexity theory
Outcomes, clinical. *See* Clinical outcomes
"Outliers," 24
Out-of-town hospital headquarters, effect of, 100–101
Outpatient capacity, 87
Outpatient care, 87, 94
Outputs and inputs, 110, 112, 128. *See also* Complexity theory
Outsourcing, 29, 31–32, 34
Overcapacity, 85, 86–87
Overorganization, 66
Ownership conversions, 126
Ownership shuffle, 9, 98, 100
Oxford, 141

P

Pacific Business Group on Health, 70
PacifiCare, 49, 141
"Painful Pursuit of a Competitive Marketplace," 17
Paracelsus, 98
"Paradigm Lost: Deconstructing the Columbia/HCA Investigation," 99
Parallel systems, effect of, 20–21
Parikh, N., 167
Passi, G., 117–118, 119
Patagonia, 54, 55

Pathological periodicities, 118
Patient accountability, 52, 122, 159, 187
Patient behavior, 79, 80, 121–123
Patient information, sharing, 148
Patient pull-through strategy, 156
Patient scheduling, integrating, obstacle to, 147
Patient-physician relationship, 101–102, 180, 196
Patients: consumers becoming, rate of, 77; importance of, 206. *See also under specific topics*
Patient's bill of rights, 47, 191
Patterning, 112, 117, 118, 119, 122, 126
Pauly, M., 126, 171
Payer alignment, 89
Payer mix, 88
Payers, third-party, 32, 51, 52, 140
Payroll deduction, 187
PCS, 136
Peeno, L., 64–65
Penalties for compliance failure, 21–22
Pension funds, protection of, 5–6
Per member per month (PMPM) payment. *See* Capitation
Perceived quality, 185, 186
Performance information, 157–158
Performance measurement, 120
Periodicities, pathological, 118
Personal charity, example of, 204
Personal gain, conflict with, 2
Perturbations, 117, 118, 120, 121
Pharmaceutical drugs. *See Drug entries*
Pharmaceutical Research and Manufacturers of America, 73, 173
Pharmacies, on-line, 136
Pharmacy cost inflation, aggregate, 155
Pharmacy price inflation, 155
Phillips, K. A., 61
"PHOs Losing Steam," 147
Physician costs, 59
Physician groups, integration of, attempts at, 7–8
Physician Hospital Organizations (PHOs), 147

Physician lobby, 56
Physician pay data, 126
Physician quality, 59
Physician-hospital integration, 7, 12, 146–147
Physician-hospital relationship, 10, 11–12, 101, 102, 103, 104, 146–148
Physician-patient relationship, 101–102, 180, 196
Physicians, 102; coddling of, 94; control over, 55, 104; involving, in decision making, 84, 101, 103; managing, 101; power of, 101, 102; younger generation of, 68. *See also under specific topics*
Plaintiffs' Legal Committee, Buckman v., 48
Playboy Enterprises, 54
Pneumonia, 81, 82
Point of service (POS) plans, 63, 156
Political interests, threat to, 183
Politicization, avoiding, 197, 198
Pollitz, K., 42, 47, 190–191
Portability. *See* Health insurance portability
Practice patterns, 124–125
Practice variations, 110
Pre-approval process, scrapping, 90
Prediction, ineffectiveness of, 113, 117, 126–127, 128
Preexisting conditions, 38, 39, 41, 47, 190
Preferred provider organizations (PPOs), 35, 140
Premiums. *See* Health insurance premiums
Prescription drugs. *See Drug entries*
Prescription refills, 133, 136, 174
Preventable deaths, 110, 111, 138
Prevention and wellness care, 55, 56, 58; economics of, 17, 67, 81, 82, 122, 169–170
Price discounts, 192
Price discrimination, 192, 193
Price regulations, 5, 188, 189, 191–193
Price sensitivity, 158
Price shopping, borderless, 188
Price stabilization, 185
Price-performance ratio, 183
Pricing: aggressive, 87; competitive, 89
Primary care, 167, 168, 169–170, 175

Primary care physicians, 90
Print advertising, 155
Print media, 46, 75, 200
Private and public system, 13, 20, 74
Private health care choices, public funding of, problem with, 23, 24
Private health insurance system, market failure of, 91
Privatization, 15, 16
Pro bono care, 166, 172, 174
Proactive charity care, 170
Product differentiation, 40
Productivity, 36, 37, 38, 82
Profiteering and insolvency, 22
Progress, meaning of, 206
Progressive companies, 30
Proprietary information technologies, 145
Providers: economic conflicts of, 51; information on, access to, 151–152; performance of, 120, 157–158; selection of, 152, 156, 157, 158, 179; self-serving nature of, 2. *See also Hospital entries; Physician entries*
Prozac, 79
Prudential, 42
Public and private system, 13, 19–20, 74
Public data sets, 158
Public funding of private health care choices, 23, 24
Public health advocates, 55
Public health promotion, desire for, 184
Pull-through strategy, 155–156
Purchasers, third-party, 51, 52, 72, 88, 140
Purchasing cooperatives, 33
Purchasing insurance coverage, 29–30, 49, 50, 187
Purchasing matrix, 88
Purchasing medical products, 100, 103
Purchasing pool, largest, 187
Purchasing power, seeking, 100

Q

Quality improvement, 32, 35–36, 80, 81
Quality measurement movement, restrictions facing, 38
Quality of care, 58, 63, 82, 185; compar-

Vladeck, B. C., 89
Voltaire, 1
Voluntary Choice Cooperatives (VCCs), 186

W

Waldholz, M., 153, 156
Walker, T., 124
Wall Street, 18, 19, 43, 117, 134; and connectivity, 137–139, 146, 161, 162; valuation by, 88, 135
Wall Street Journal, 21, 33, 62, 75, 110, 114, 156, 181
Wal-Mart, 54
Ware, J., Jr., 60
Warnock, A., III, 133
Wartime pay freeze, 1, 3
Washington Post, 129
Web sites, consumer health care, 153
Web site sharing, 147, 148
Web-based computing. *See* Internet connectivity; Internet-based computing
Web-based direct-to-consumer (DTC) advertising, 155–156

Web-based insurer, 187
Web-based medical claims processing, 45, 141–142, 144
Web-based purchasing, 49, 50
WebMD, 139, 140, 146, 153, 157; funding method of, 162–163; and medical claims processing, 141, 142, 143, 144, 145; rise and fall of, 135–137
Wechsler, J., 6, 42
Wellness care. *See* Prevention and wellness care
Wellpoint, 49, 141
West, B. J., 116
Winslow, R., 75
Working capital, seeking, 100
Workplace gains, 36–37, 38, 82
World War II, 1, 3, 28

X

Xcare.net, 139

Y

Y2K, 138